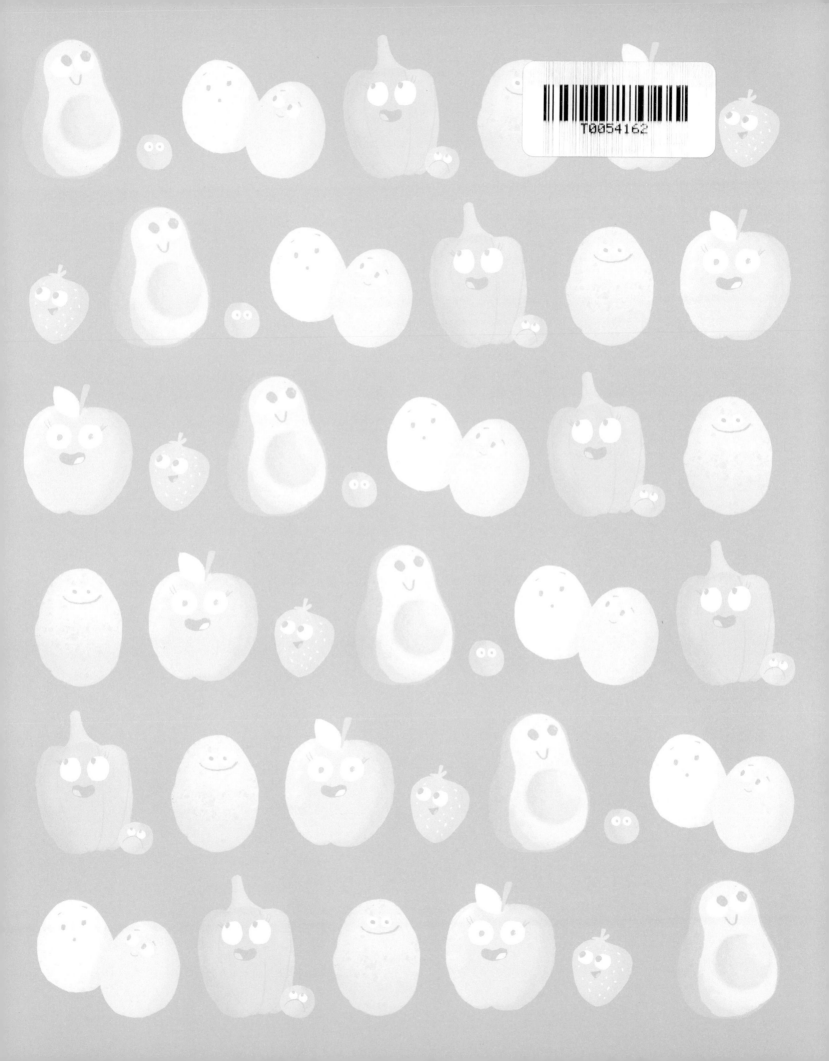

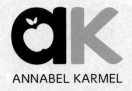

ANNABEL KARMEL

Annabel Karmel

Cook my first book

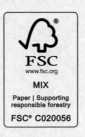

Published in 2023 by Welbeck Children's
An Imprint of Welbeck Children's Limited,
part of the Welbeck Publishing Group
Offices in: London - 20 Mortimer Street, London W1T 3JW &
Sydney - Level 17, 207 Kent St, Sydney NSW 2000 Australia
www.welbeckpublishing.com

A CIP catalogue record for this book is available
from the British Library.

ISBN: 978 1 78312 988 1

Printed in Heshan, China

10 9 8 7 6 5 4 3 2 1

Editor: Joff Brown
Design Manager: Matt Drew
Illustration: Alex Willmore
Ingredients illustrations: Bryony Clarkson
Photography: Ant Duncan
Models: Freya, Riley, Madeleine, Lincoln, Cassius,
Jake, Amaria, Noa, Leimai, Isabella, Margot, William,
Tiana, Hunter, Amelia and Teddy
Props: Tamsin Weston
Food stylist: Holly Cowgill
Production: Melanie Robertson

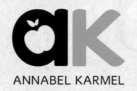

ANNABEL KARMEL

Annabel Karmel

Cookbook my first

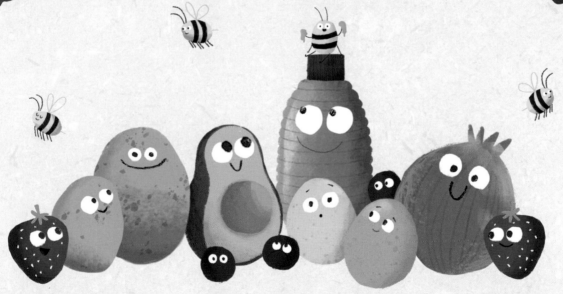

Fun, simple recipes all kids will love

Illustrated by **Alex Willmore**

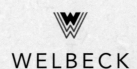

WELBECK

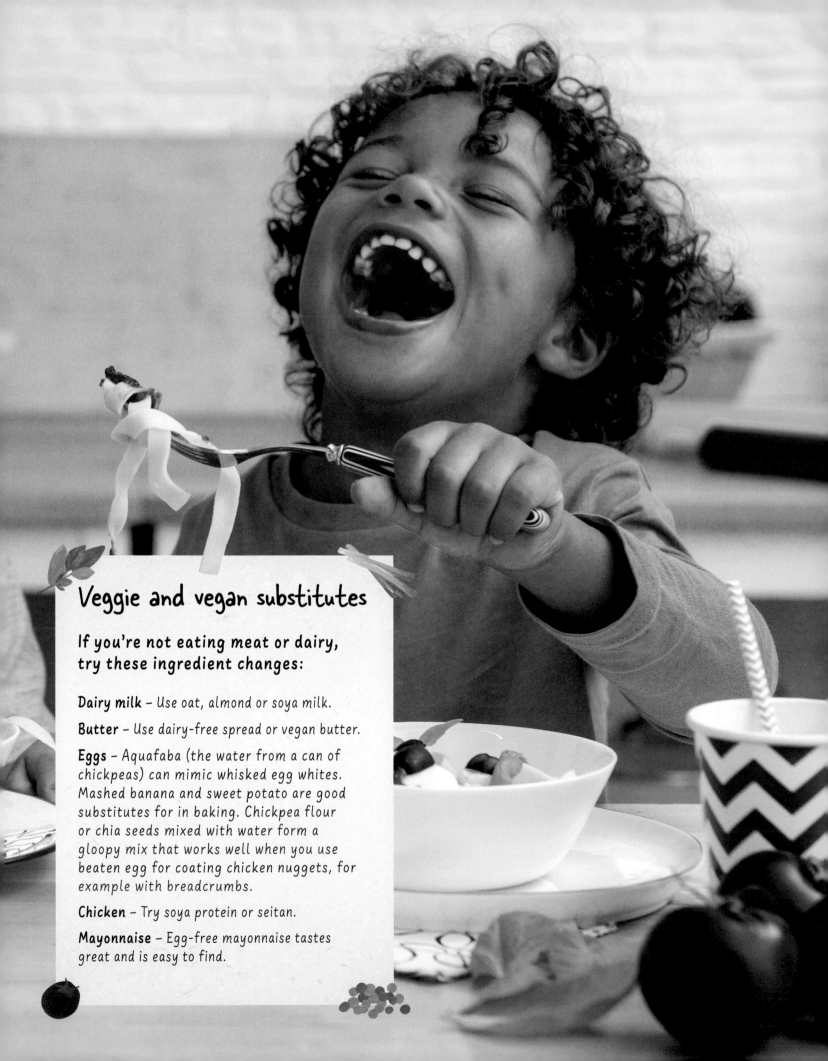

Veggie and vegan substitutes

If you're not eating meat or dairy, try these ingredient changes:

Dairy milk – Use oat, almond or soya milk.

Butter – Use dairy-free spread or vegan butter.

Eggs – Aquafaba (the water from a can of chickpeas) can mimic whisked egg whites. Mashed banana and sweet potato are good substitutes for in baking. Chickpea flour or chia seeds mixed with water form a gloopy mix that works well when you use beaten egg for coating chicken nuggets, for example with breadcrumbs.

Chicken – Try soya protein or seitan.

Mayonnaise – Egg-free mayonnaise tastes great and is easy to find.

Inside this book...

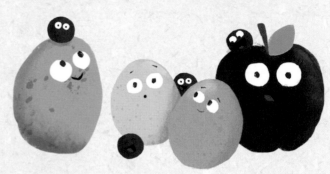

Brighten your mornings with yoghurt pancakes, a croissant crab, and more!

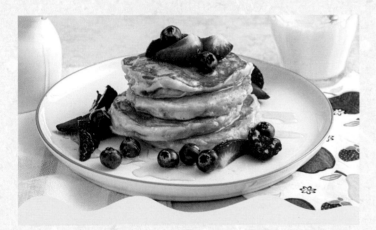

Why reach for a packet when you can make caterpillar sandwiches and monster pizza?

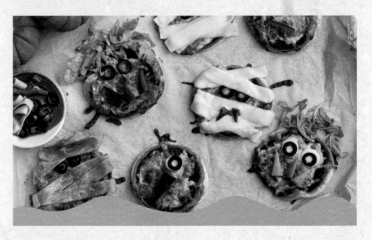

Cute pasta faces and mini beef burgers make main meals fun again.

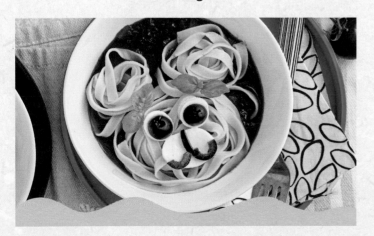

All kinds of yummy sweet treats, from teddy bear cupcakes to Oreo brownies.

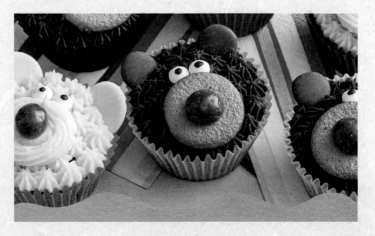

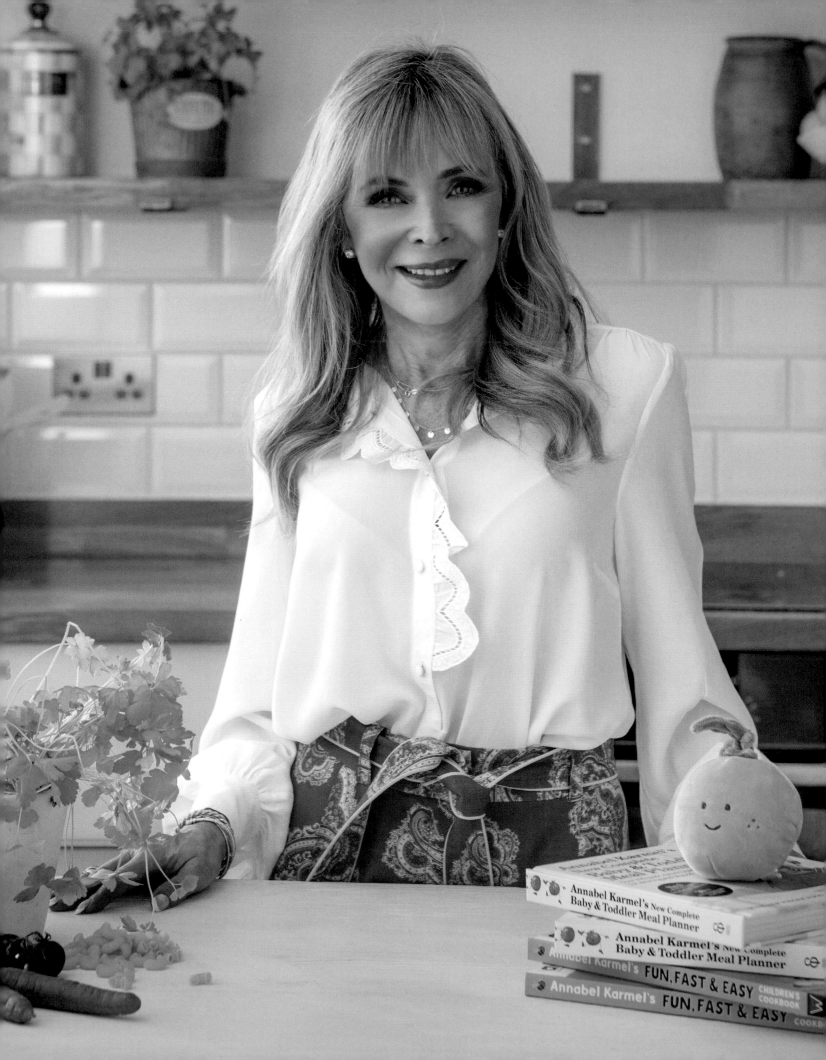

Introduction
(A little note to grown-ups!)

There really is something quite magical about cooking with kids. As a child, I can remember clambering up to the kitchen counter on my little white chair, putting on my mum's oversized apron and eagerly stirring and measuring. Licking the spoon was always the best part!

And when my three children were toddlers, I got them cooking too. I sometimes needed more than a pinch of patience with my pint-sized helpers. But the kitchen was (and still is) the place where we had fun, giggles, got a bit messy, and made mountains of memories!

Cooking is one of the most valuable skills we can teach children, and it's never too early to learn. There's a lot of "I want to do it myself" when they start out, which is a wonderful thing because with a bit of practice, they really will be able to do it all by themselves!

I got to a point where my three children under 6 were taking the reins on Friday night dinner. It didn't always unfold the way I'd imagined, but I'll never forget the expression on their little faces when they presented me with their cooking conquests. They were bursting with pride and self-confidence.

My brand new cookbook is the perfect inroad to sparking a lifelong love of food and cooking. Each simple recipe includes step-by-step instructions and fun illustrations. They'll get to practice all kinds of basic skills such as mixing, rolling, stirring, squeezing, cutting and measuring. You won't believe how satisfying they'll find cracking eggs and kneading dough!

I've packed in a rainbow of ingredients for your budding chefs to explore, most of which you'll already have at home. From power-packed breakfasts and dinner winners to healthy snacks and little treats, my recipes will bring the whole family together.

Happy cooking!

Things you can do

Here's a list of some of the things **YOU** can do to help in the kitchen.

You'll still need a grown-up's help to deal with anything hot or sharp, but there's plenty of ways to get involved in every recipe. **Tick the things you can do!**

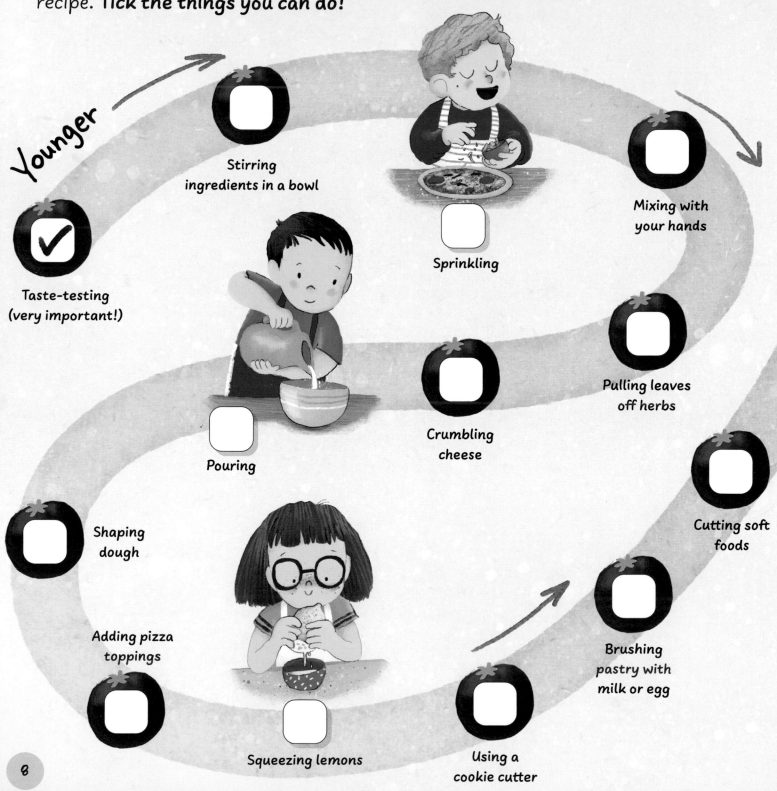

Younger

Taste-testing
(very important!)

Stirring
ingredients in a bowl

Sprinkling

Mixing with
your hands

Pouring

Crumbling
cheese

Pulling leaves
off herbs

Cutting soft
foods

Shaping
dough

Adding pizza
toppings

Squeezing lemons

Using a
cookie cutter

Brushing
pastry with
milk or egg

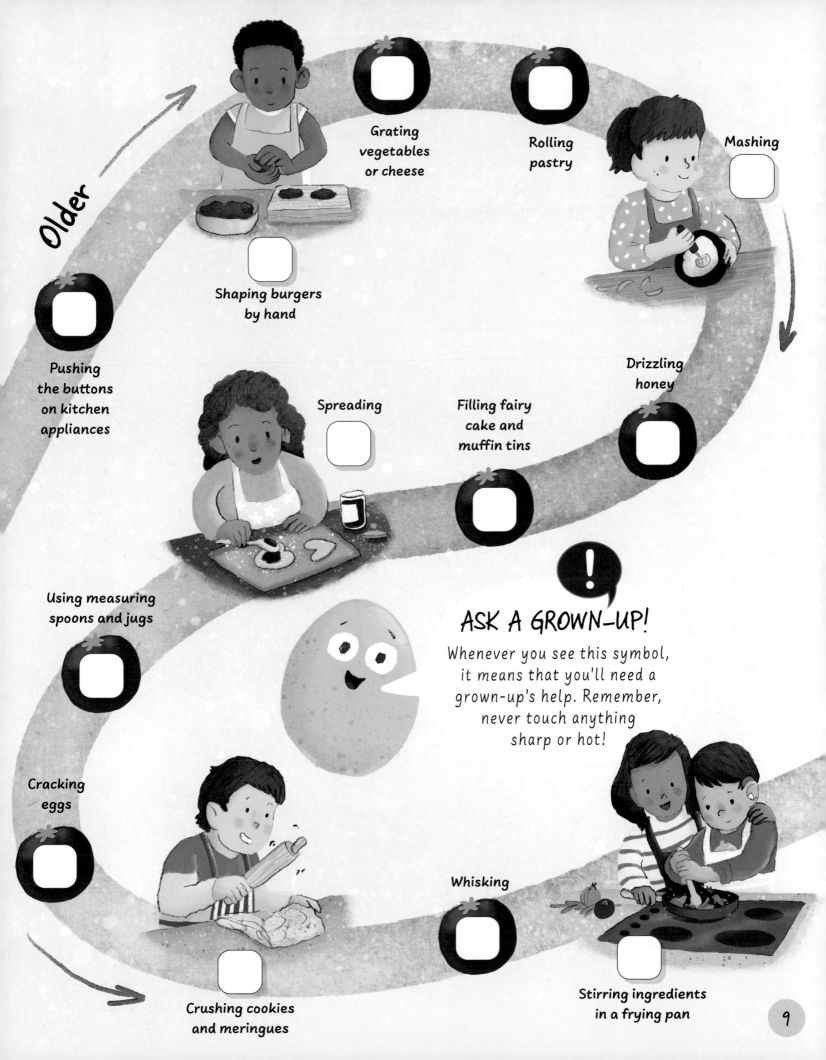

Older

Grating
vegetables
or cheese

Rolling
pastry

Mashing

Shaping burgers
by hand

Pushing
the buttons
on kitchen
appliances

Spreading

Filling fairy
cake and
muffin tins

Drizzling
honey

Using measuring
spoons and jugs

!

ASK A GROWN-UP!

Whenever you see this symbol,
it means that you'll need a
grown-up's help. Remember,
never touch anything
sharp or hot!

Cracking
eggs

Whisking

Crushing cookies
and meringues

Stirring ingredients
in a frying pan

9

Things you need

You don't need to have all of this equipment to make the recipes in this book, but if you do, it will help.

Frying pan
The big flat one! It's perfect for cooking small or thin things.

Saucepan
The deep one! This is great for making sauces, soups, and mashed potatoes.

Baking paper
You can put this in the oven – food won't stick to it.

Cling film
Great for wrapping dough or pastry while it's chilling.

Measuring spoons
A tablespoon is bigger than a teaspoon. Make sure you use the right one!

Garlic Press
Makes crushing bulbs of garlic super easy.

Sieve/colander
The one with the holes in! Use a big one for draining pasta or rice and a mini one for dusting cookies with sugar.

Cookie cutters
Press these into dough with the sharp end down.

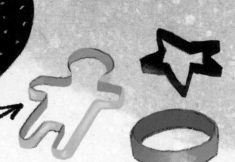

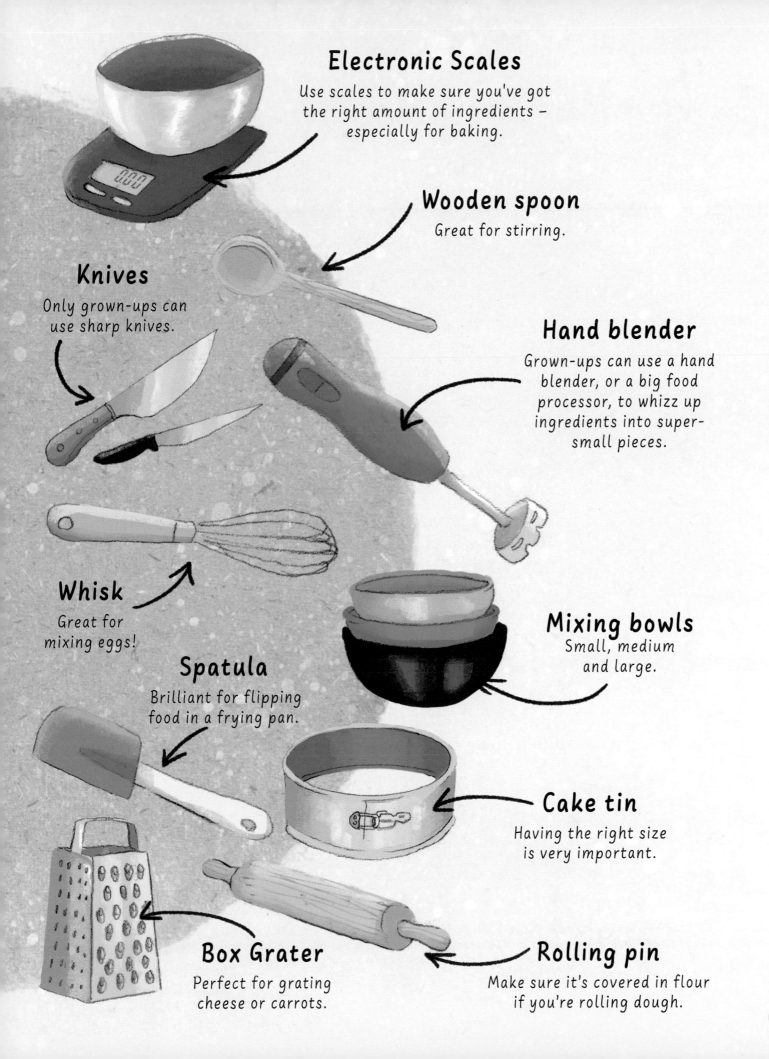

Electronic Scales
Use scales to make sure you've got the right amount of ingredients – especially for baking.

Wooden spoon
Great for stirring.

Knives
Only grown-ups can use sharp knives.

Hand blender
Grown-ups can use a hand blender, or a big food processor, to whizz up ingredients into super-small pieces.

Whisk
Great for mixing eggs!

Mixing bowls
Small, medium and large.

Spatula
Brilliant for flipping food in a frying pan.

Cake tin
Having the right size is very important.

Box Grater
Perfect for grating cheese or carrots.

Rolling pin
Make sure it's covered in flour if you're rolling dough.

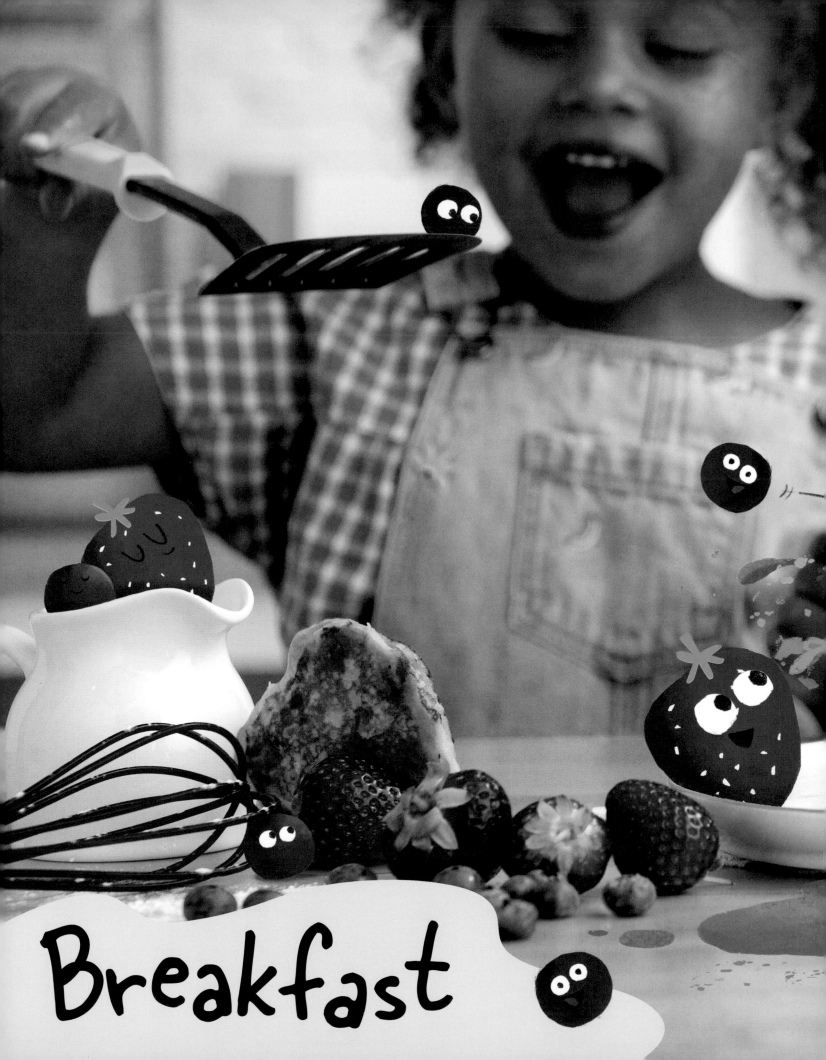

Breakfast

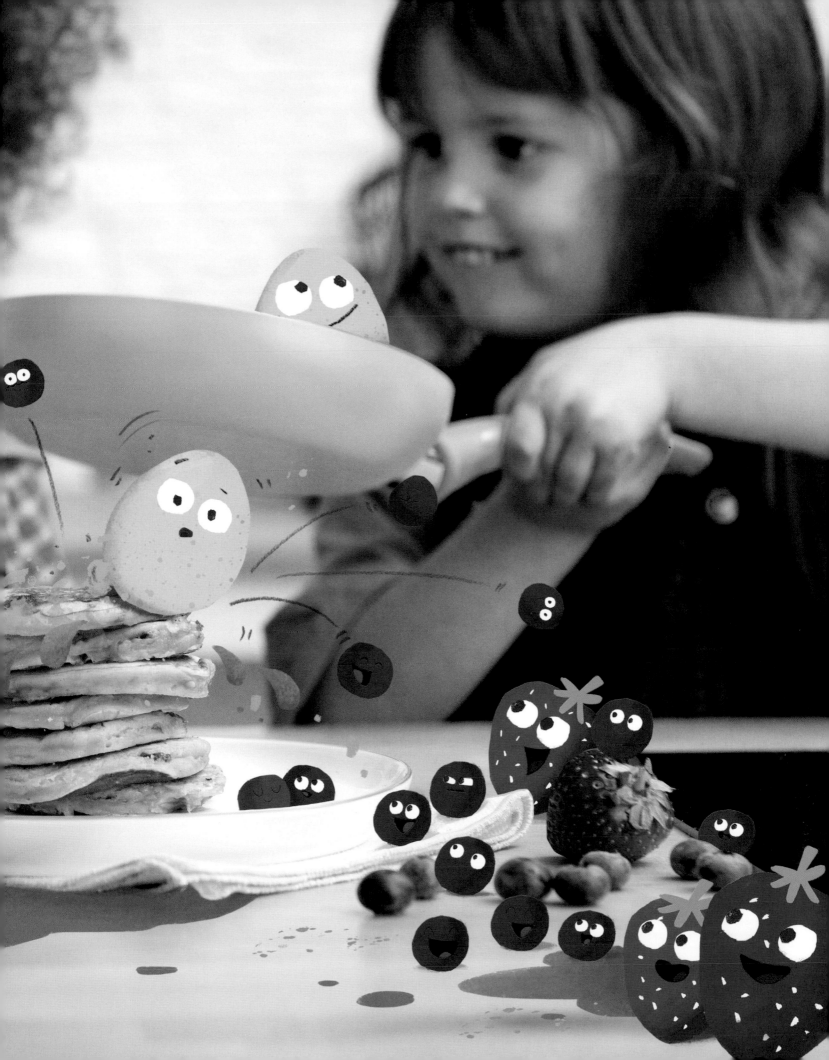

Animal porridge

Healthy oats are a great way to start your day – fruity animals make it even more fun!

You will need

 80g (1 cup) porridge oats

 500ml (2 cups) milk of your choice – dairy, oat, almond or soy are all great

For the bunny

 1 red apple

 blueberries

 chocolate chips

 chocolate icing pen

For the chick

 ½ ripe mango, diced

 strawberries

 blueberries

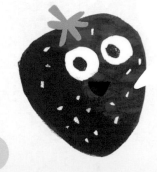

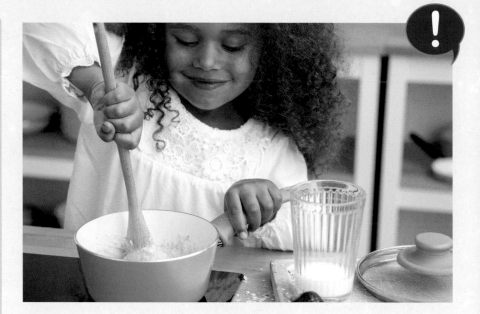

1 Make the porridge by heating the oats and the milk in a saucepan until it just boils.

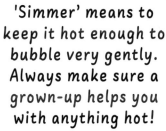
'Simmer' means to keep it hot enough to bubble very gently. Always make sure a grown-up helps you with anything hot!

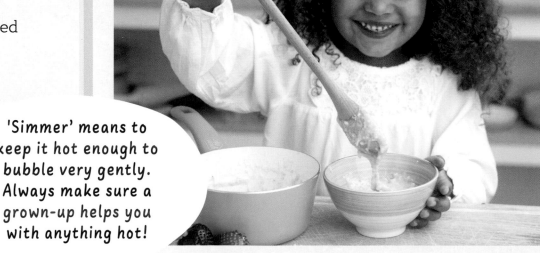

2 Quick! Reduce the heat so it doesn't boil over. Simmer for 4 minutes. When it's ready, spoon into two bowls.

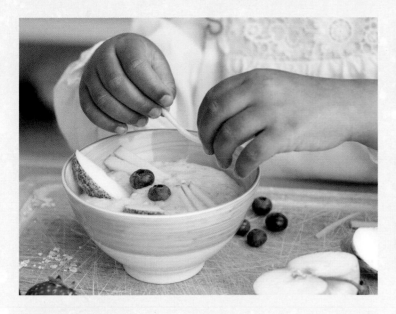
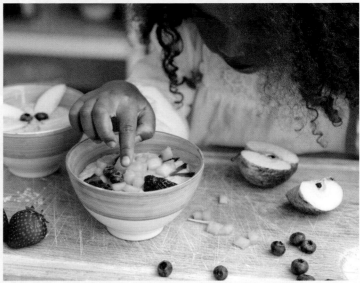

3 Make the bunny by adding two apple wedges for the ears, two blueberries for the eyes and a chocolate chip for the nose. Add a mouth using the chocolate icing pen.

4 For the chick, arrange the diced mango in two circles on the porridge. Add two strawberry slices for the wings and blueberries for the eyes. Make the legs and comb out of strawberries.

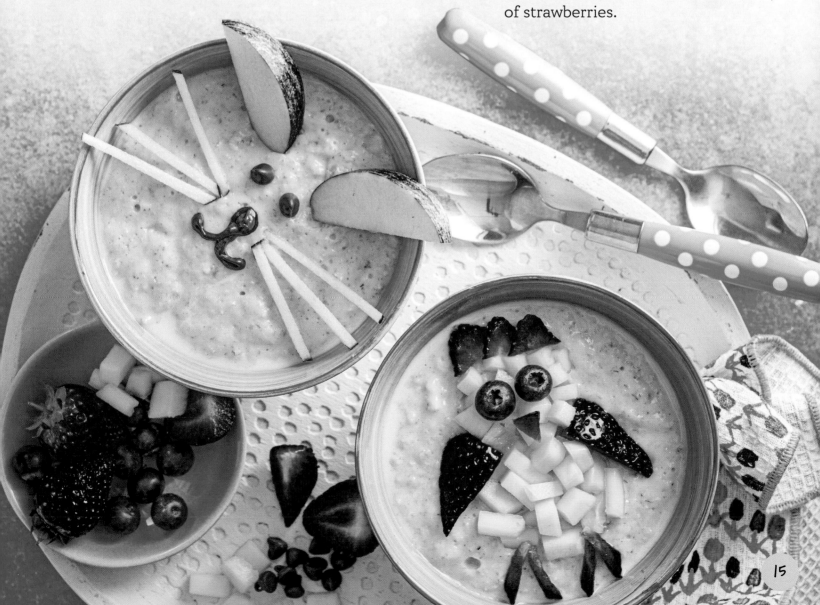

Makes
15

Veggie

Prep time
10 mins

Cook time
3 mins

Yoghurt pancakes
with banana, apple and sultana

You'll love making these fluffy, puffy pancakes, and topping them with all kinds of fruit.

You will need

 1 egg, beaten

 100g (1 cup) self-raising flour

 75ml (⅓ cup) milk

 150g (6-oz cup) Greek yoghurt

 1 large overripe banana, mashed

 1 small apple, peeled and grated

 50g (⅓ cup) sultanas

 sunflower oil

 honey

 fruit of your choice to serve - I love blueberries and strawberries!

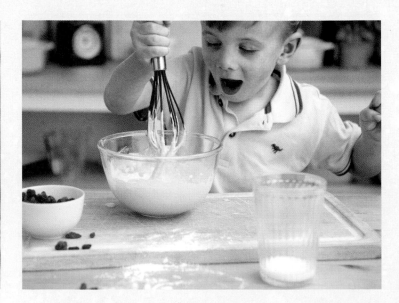

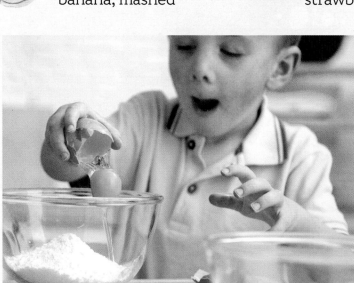

1 Measure the egg, flour, milk, yoghurt, banana and apple into a bowl.

2 Whisk until smooth, then add the sultanas.

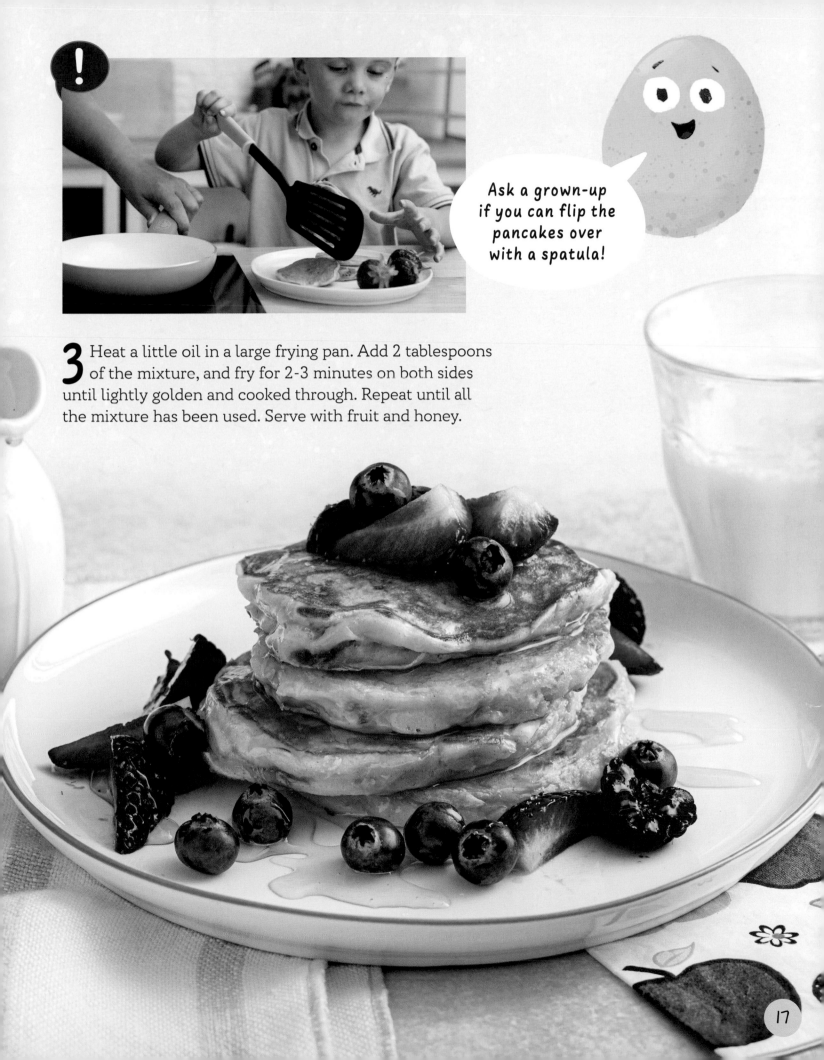

Ask a grown-up if you can flip the pancakes over with a spatula!

3 Heat a little oil in a large frying pan. Add 2 tablespoons of the mixture, and fry for 2-3 minutes on both sides until lightly golden and cooked through. Repeat until all the mixture has been used. Serve with fruit and honey.

Croissant crab

Turn breakfast into a day at the beach with this deliciously fruity crab creation!

You will need

 1 croissant

 3 large strawberries

 ½ banana

 2 blueberries

 cocktail sticks

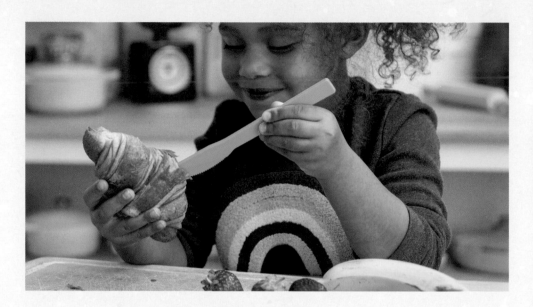

1 Put the croissant onto a board. Make a cut in one side of the croissant to make the crab's mouth.

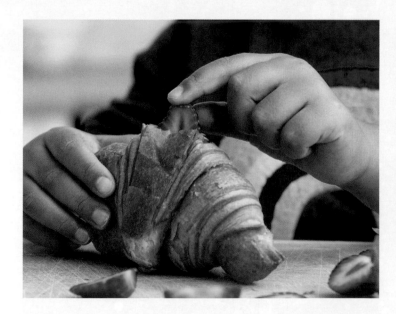

2 Slice one strawberry in half and insert into the gap to make a tongue.

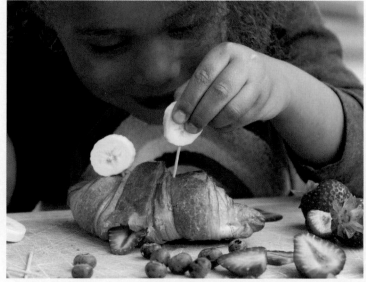

3 Slice the banana into rounds. Insert a cocktail stick and add to the croissant to make the eyes.

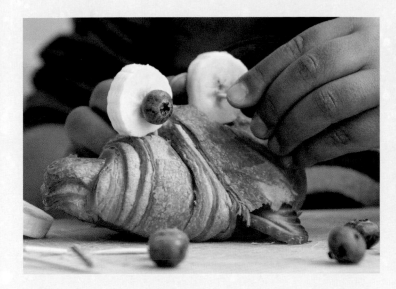

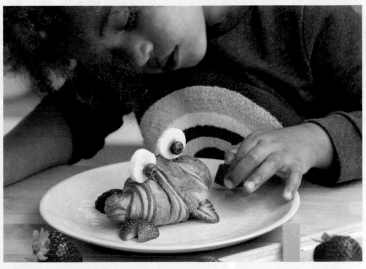

4 Snap a cocktail stick in half and place a blueberry on each one. Insert the blueberries in the centre of the banana to make the eyeballs.

5 Halve the remaining strawberries, and cut out a small triangle at the ends for the claws and legs. Remember to take all the cocktail sticks out before eating!

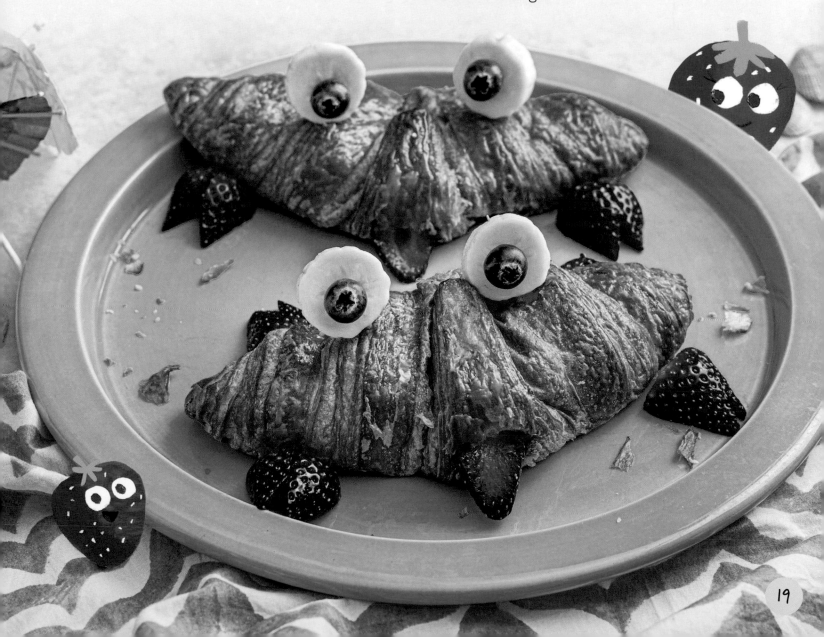

Dippy egg with Marmite and cheese fingers

Jazz up a dippy egg with some funky toast fingers!

You will need

  2 large eggs

  2 heaped teaspoons of Marmite

2 slices of white bread

50g (about 1/2 cup) Cheddar cheese, grated

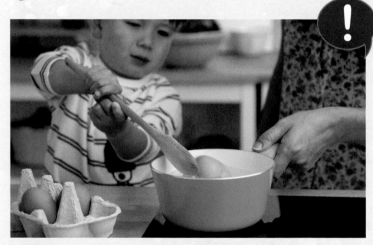

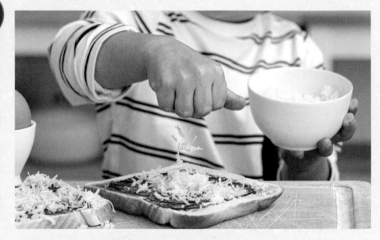

1 Bring a saucepan of water to the boil. Ask an adult to put the eggs onto spoons and gently lower into the water. Boil for 6 minutes. Drain and place in eggcups.

2 Meanwhile, preheat the grill, and toast the bread on both sides. Spread thinly with Marmite and sprinkle with cheese. Put back under the grill to melt the cheese. Slice into fingers and serve.

Scrambled eggs with ham and cheese

This simple, comforting recipe is fun and easy to make.

You will need

  2 large eggs

 2 tablespoons milk

knob of butter

 1 slice of ham, chopped

20g (3 tablespoons) Cheddar cheese, grated

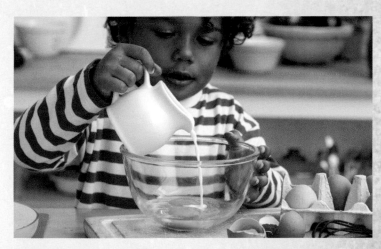

1 Break the eggs into a bowl. Add the milk and beat together. Meanwhile, melt the butter in a small frying pan.

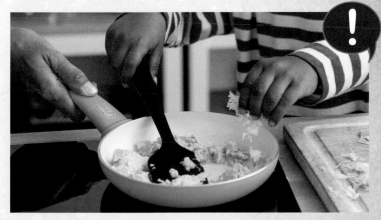

2 Add the eggs and stir over a medium heat until just set. Add the ham and cheese and gently fold into the eggs.

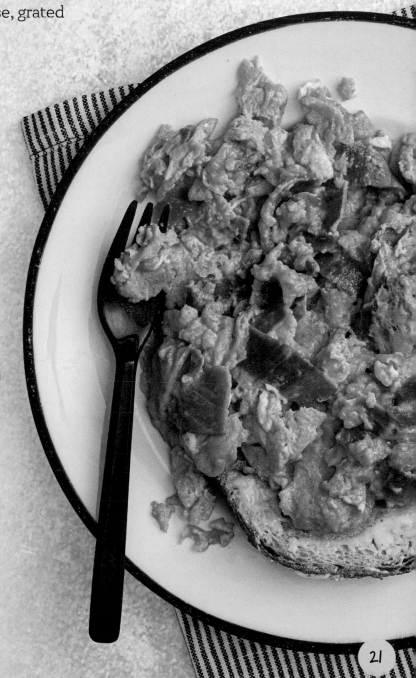

Egg in a hole

You've had eggs on toast, but how about eggs IN toast?

You will need

 knob of butter

 1 teaspoon sunflower oil

 1 slice white bread

 1 large egg

Equipment
Round cookie cutter

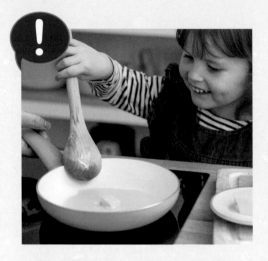

1 Heat the butter and oil in a medium-size frying pan.

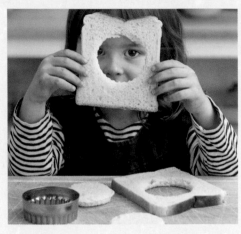

2 Put the bread onto a board. Use a cutter to stamp out a circle from the centre of the bread. Put the bread into the frying pan and fry for 2 minutes until golden.

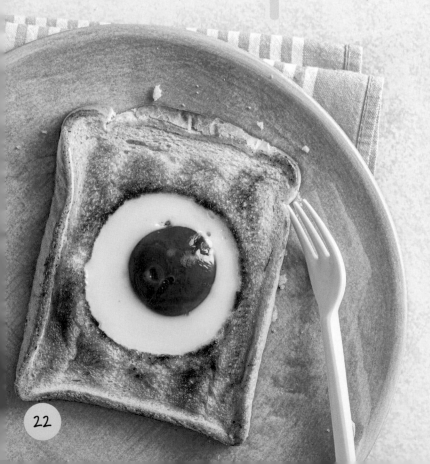

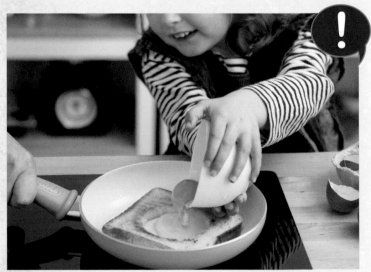

3 Turn over. Crack the egg into a bowl then carefully tip into the hole. Cover with a lid, and cook for 3-4 minutes until the egg is set.

Baked frittata

This omelette makes a hearty breakfast or an easy lunch.

You will need

 200g (7 oz) new potatoes

 6 large eggs

 2 tablespoons milk

 200g (7 oz) cherry tomatoes, quartered

 25g (3 tablespoons) frozen peas

 4 spring onions, sliced

 2 tablespoons basil

 75g (⅔ cup) Parmesan cheese, grated

1 Preheat the oven to 180°C (350°F) Fan. Grease a medium oven-proof saucepan with butter.

2 Cook the potatoes in boiling salted water for 12 minutes until tender. Drain well and cut into slices.

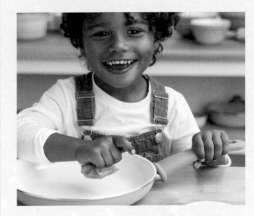

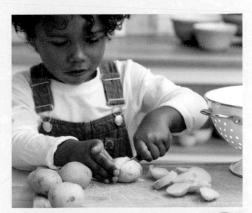

3 Beat the eggs and milk together in a mixing bowl. Add the potatoes, tomatoes, peas, onions, basil and cheese. Pour into the saucepan. Bake for 30 minutes until set and lightly golden brown.

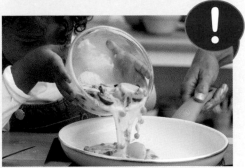

Equipment
Oven-proof saucepan

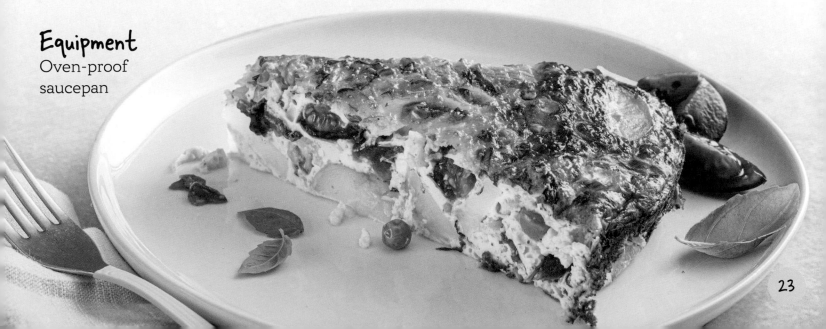

23

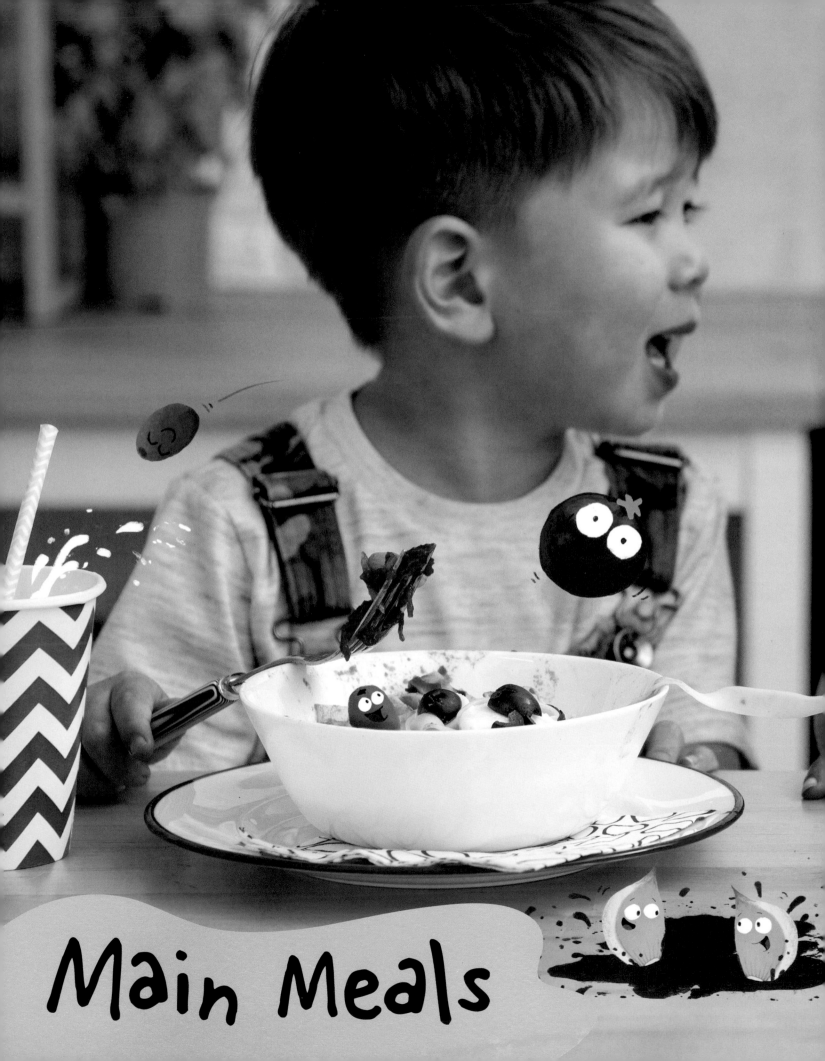

Main Meals

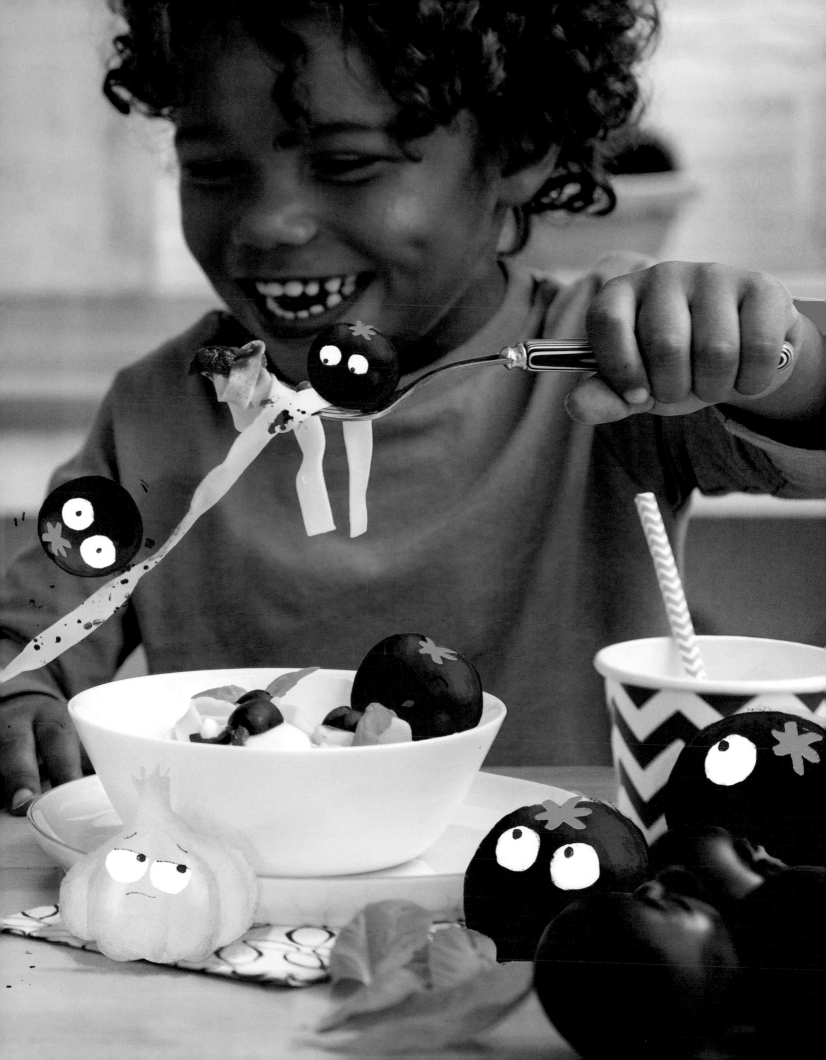

Sticky chicken with sweet potato fries

Nobody can resist this sweet, sticky chicken, especially with healthy baked fries.

You will need

  3 tablespoons ketchup

 3 tablespoons soy sauce

 2 tablespoons honey

 2 cloves of garlic, crushed

500g (18 oz) boneless chicken thighs, sliced into strips

 3 medium sweet potatoes, scrubbed

 2 tablespoons sunflower oil

 1 teaspoon chopped thyme

 3 tablespoons semolina

Equipment
Baking tray, baking paper

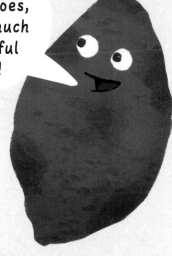

Who needs regular potatoes, when I'm so much more colourful and tasty!

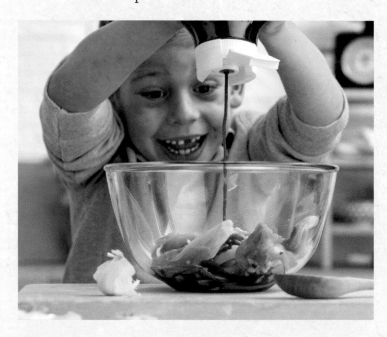

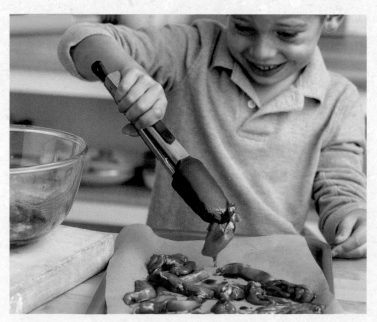

1 Put the chicken into a medium mixing bowl. Add the ketchup, soy, honey and garlic, and mix together to coat the chicken.

2 Leave for 30 minutes, then arrange on a baking tray lined with baking paper. Preheat the oven to 200°C (400°F) Fan.

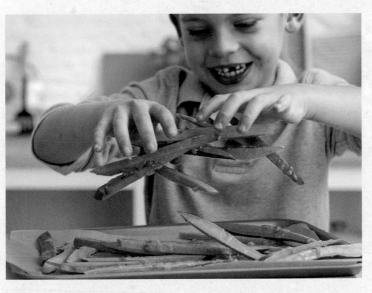

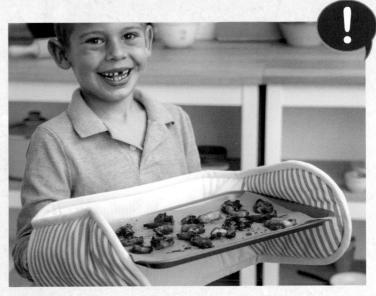

3 Slice the sweet potatoes into thin chip shapes. Place on a baking sheet lined with baking paper. Add the oil and thyme. Season with salt and pepper, and coat with semolina to make them crispy. Mix everything up with your hands. Spread out on the baking sheet in a single layer.

4 Put both baking sheets into the oven. Cook for about 25 minutes, until the chicken is cooked and golden brown and the fries are lightly golden and cooked through.

Swap it!

To make this recipe veggie, use meat-free strips instead of chicken.

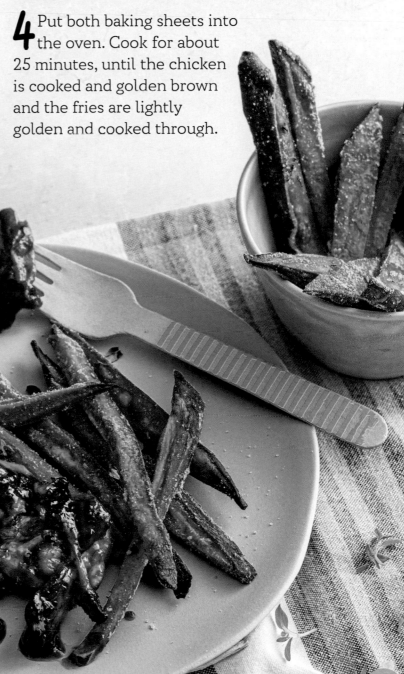

Serves
4–6

Veggie

Prep time
20mins

Cooking
1hr

Funny face baked potatoes

Who can make the funniest face for these potato heads?

You will need

 4 baking potatoes, scrubbed

 2 tablespoons mayonnaise

 25g (¼ cup) Cheddar cheese, grated

 2 spring onions, chopped

 145g (5 oz) tin tuna, drained

For decoration

 ½ red pepper

 ½ yellow pepper

 Mozzarella

 black olives

 peas, cooked

 1 carrot, grated

 cherry tomatoes

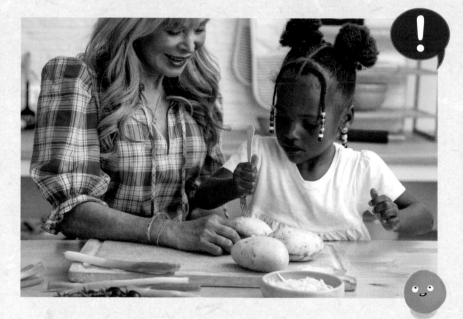

1 Preheat the oven to 180°C (350°F) Fan. Prick the potatoes. Bake in the oven for 45 minutes–1 hour, until the potatoes are soft and the skins are golden.

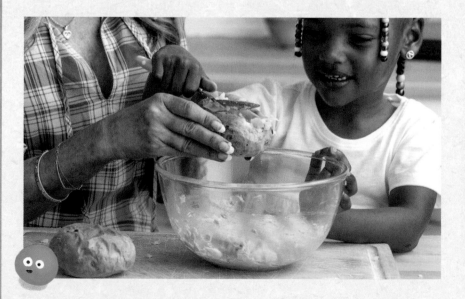

2 Put the mayo, cheese, spring onion and tuna into a bowl. Make a hole on one side of the potato. Scoop out the cooked potato, and mix it in.

28

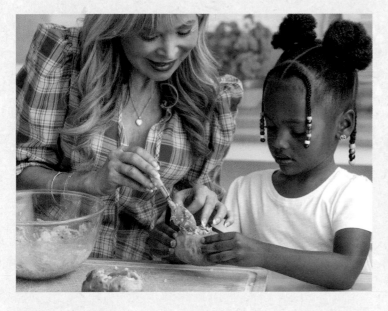

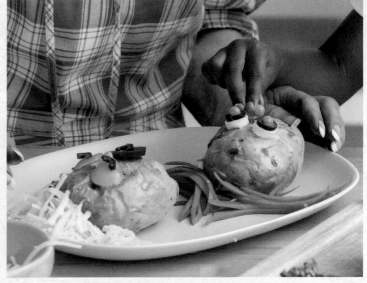

3 Mix well and season with salt and pepper. Spoon the mashed mixture back into the potato shells.

4 Turn upside down. Decorate the potatoes by making funny faces. Add slices of peppers, cheese, olives, peas, carrot and tomatoes for the eyes, mouths and hair.

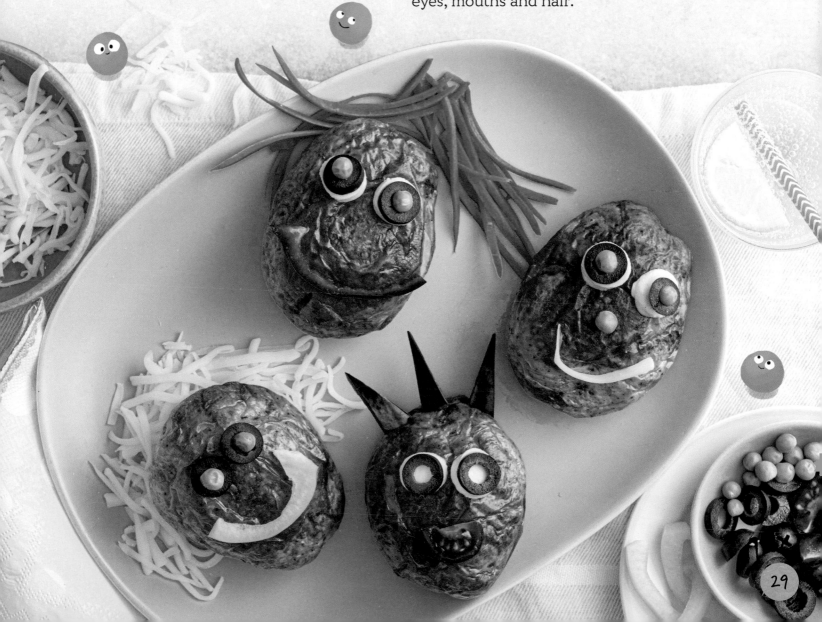

Smoky chicken and rice

A warming recipe that's easy to cook, and even easier to eat!

You will need

 2 tablespoons sunflower oil

 1 onion, chopped

 1 small red pepper, diced

 1 small carrot, diced

 2 cloves garlic, crushed

 1 teaspoon sweet smoked paprika

 200g (1 cup) long grain rice

 200ml (just over ¾ cup) passata

 500ml (2 cups) chicken stock

 1 teaspoon thyme, chopped

 75g (½ cup) peas

 6 cherry tomatoes, quartered

 150g (5 oz) cooked chicken breast, diced

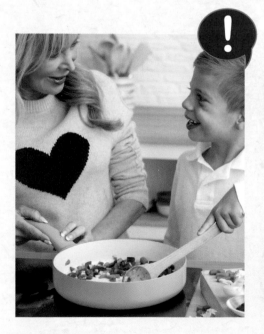

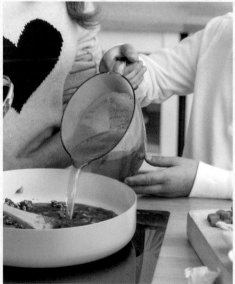

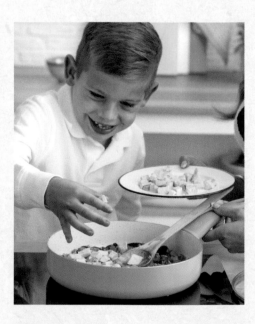

1 Heat the oil to a medium heat in a sauté pan. Add the onion, pepper and carrot, and fry for a few minutes.

2 Add the garlic and fry for 10 seconds. Add the paprika, rice, passata, stock and thyme. Cover with a lid, bring to the boil, and simmer for 15 minutes.

3 Remove the lid and add the peas, tomatoes and chicken. Simmer for 2-3 minutes. Serve as soon as it's cooked.

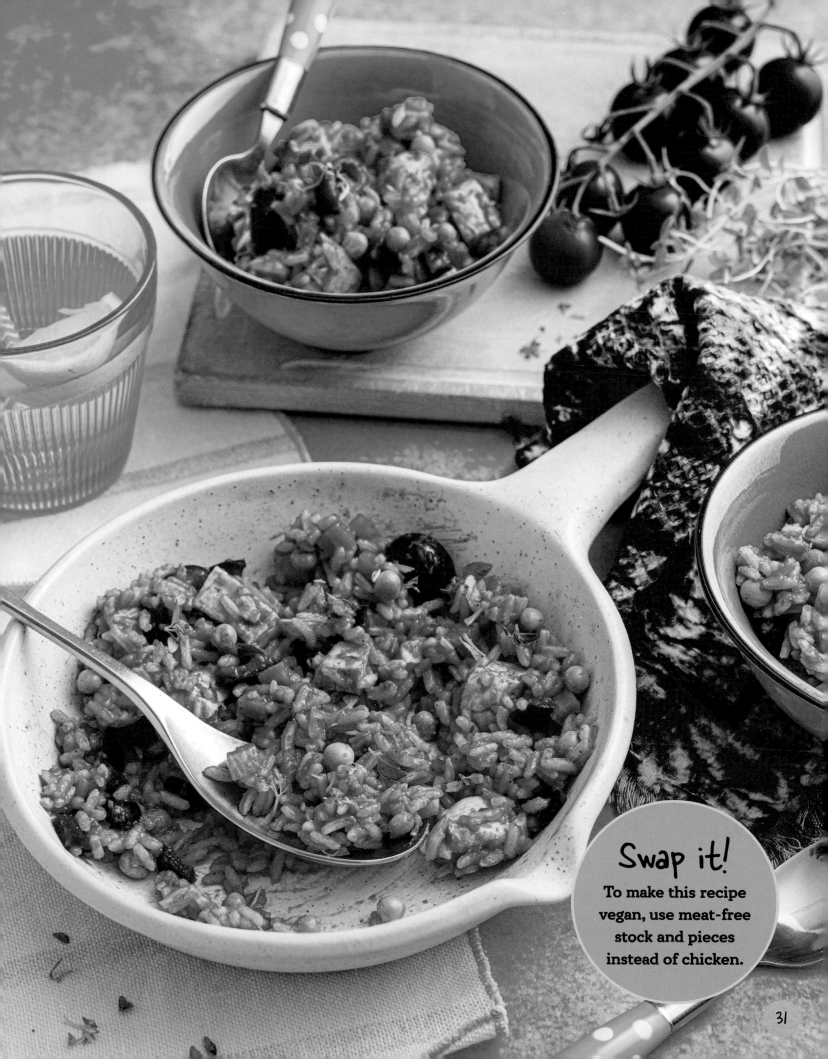

Swap it!
To make this recipe
vegan, use meat-free
stock and pieces
instead of chicken.

Serves
4

Veggie

Prep time
15mins

Cooking
20mins

Teddy bear tomato pasta

Who knew that pasta could look so cute... and tasty!

You will need

 2 tablespoons olive oil

 1 onion, chopped finely

 2 cloves garlic, crushed

 2 x 400g (14 oz) cans chopped tomatoes

 2 tablespoons tomato purée

 dash of sugar

 300g (11 oz) fresh tagliatelle pasta

 Mozzarella ball

 pitted black olives

 basil

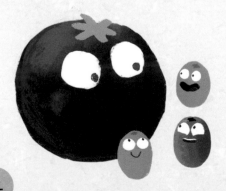

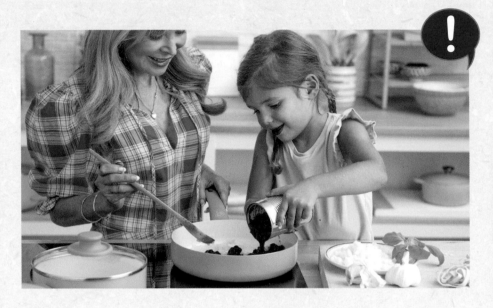

1 Heat the oil in a large saucepan. Add the onion and garlic and fry for 5 minutes. Add the chopped tomatoes and purée. Simmer for 15 minutes, until the sauce has reduced to a thick consistency. Add the sugar, and season well.

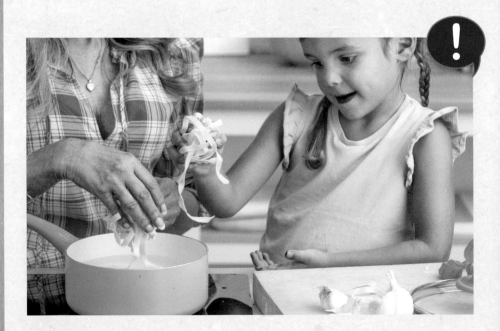

2 Cook the pasta in boiling water according to the packet instructions, then drain.

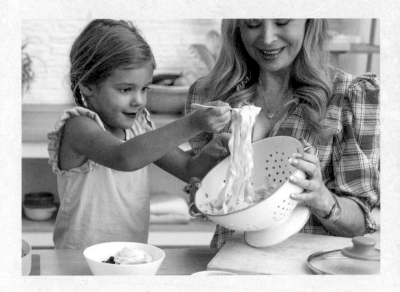

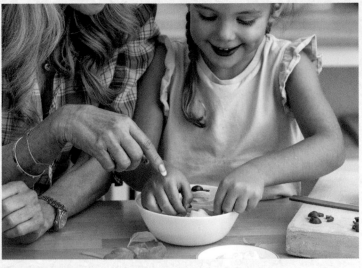

3 Put the tomato sauce into a bowl. Shape the pasta into a ball and place it on top to make the bear's face. Make two smaller balls and place on top to make the ears. Put two small Mozzarella balls on for the eyes.

4 Add slices of olives for the pupils. Use a round slice of Mozzarella for the face, and add olives for the nose and mouth. Garnish with basil leaves for a stylish finish!

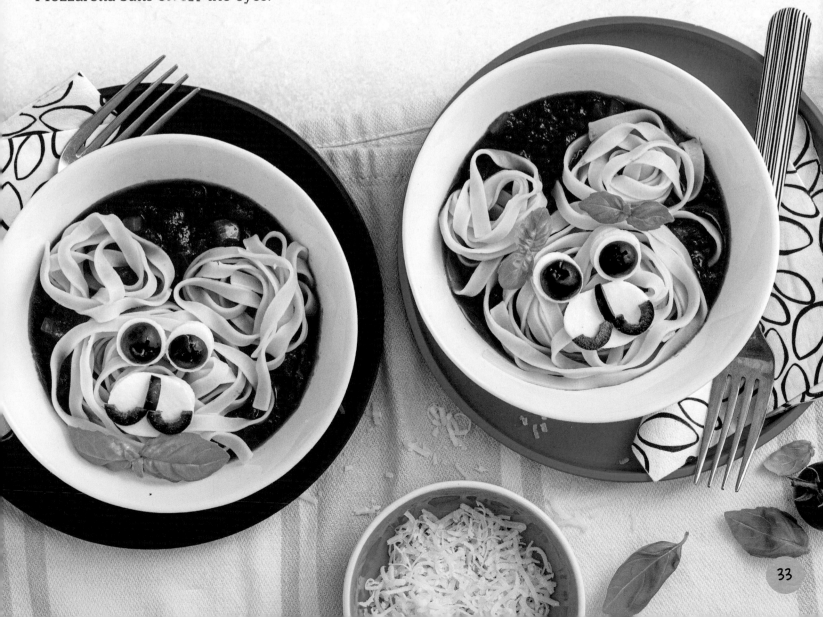

Mini beef burgers

Hidden veggies and apple makes these burgers extra yummy.

You will need

 ½ carrot, peeled and grated

 ½ onion, chopped

 ½ apple, peeled and grated

30g (¼ cup) panko breadcrumbs

 2 tablespoons basil, chopped

 2 teaspoons thyme, chopped

350g (12 oz) lean mince beef

 a few drops of Worcestershire sauce

 small soft white buns

 1 tomato, sliced

 Cheddar cheese, sliced

 lettuce

Equipment
Food processor

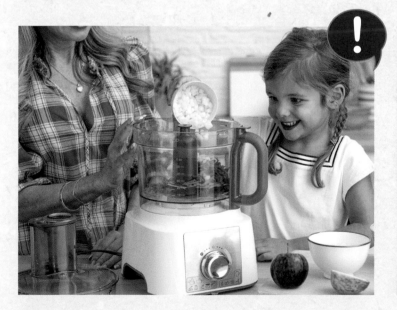

1 Measure the carrot, onion and apple into a food processor.

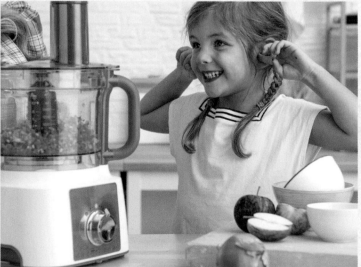

2 Whizz until the vegetables are finely chopped. Add the remaining ingredients, and season. Whiz until the mixture comes together.

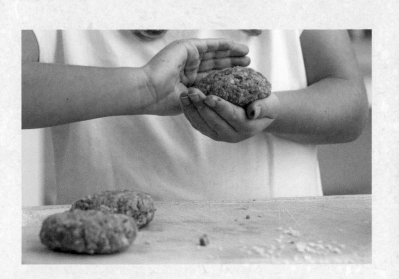

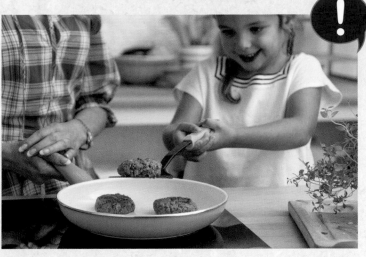

3 Shape into 10 small burgers. Now heat a little oil in a large frying pan. Add the burgers.

4 Fry for 3-4 minutes each side until golden brown and cooked through. Serve in buns with cheese, lettuce and tomato.

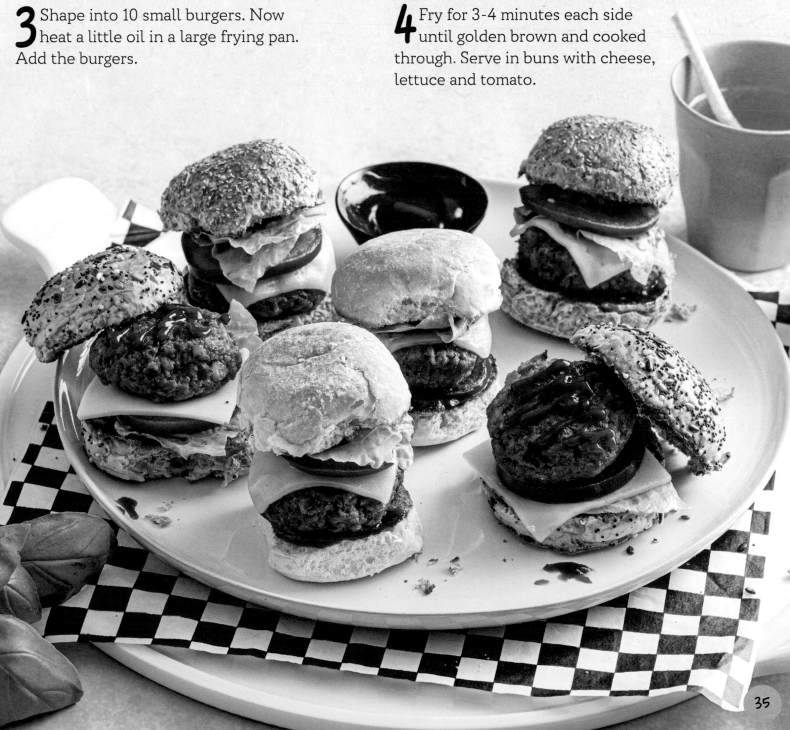

Creamy chicken soup

This creamy, comforting soup is a children's favourite.

You will need

 25g (1 oz) baby pasta shells

 25g (2 tablespoons) butter

 1 tablespoon sunflower oil

 1 onion, chopped finely

 1 medium carrot, peeled and diced

 1 small stick celery, diced finely

 100g (4 oz) butternut squash, peeled and diced

 25g (¼ cup) plain flour

 600ml (2 ½ cups) chicken stock

 40g (¼ cup) sweetcorn

 50g (2 oz) cooked chicken breast, diced

 2-3 tablespoons double cream

 1 teaspoon thyme, chopped

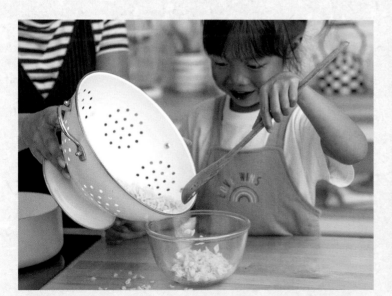

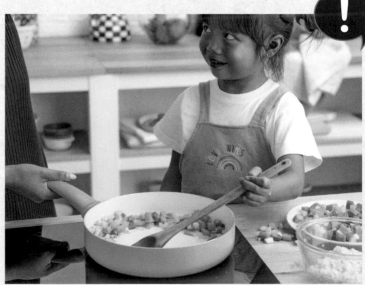

1 Cook the pasta in boiling water according to the packet instructions, then drain.

2 Melt the butter with the oil in a pan. Add the onion, carrot, celery and squash.

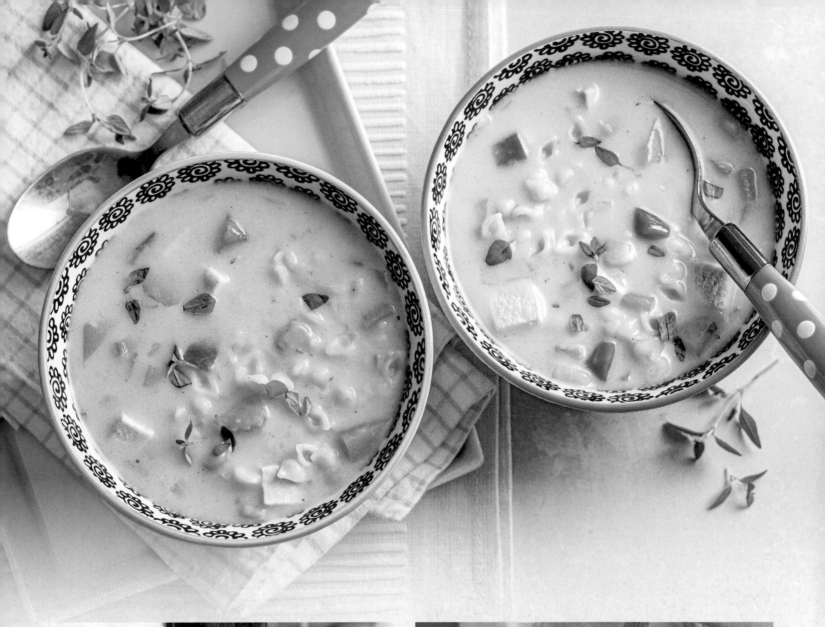

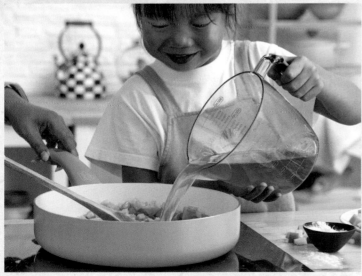

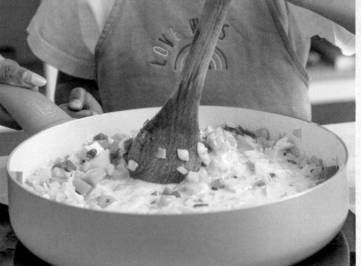

3 Stir over the heat for 4-5 minutes. Sprinkle in the flour, then slowly pour in the stock, stirring until smooth.

4 Bring up to the boil. Cover and simmer for 10 minutes. Add the sweetcorn, chicken, cream, thyme and cooked pasta. Gently simmer for 5 minutes.

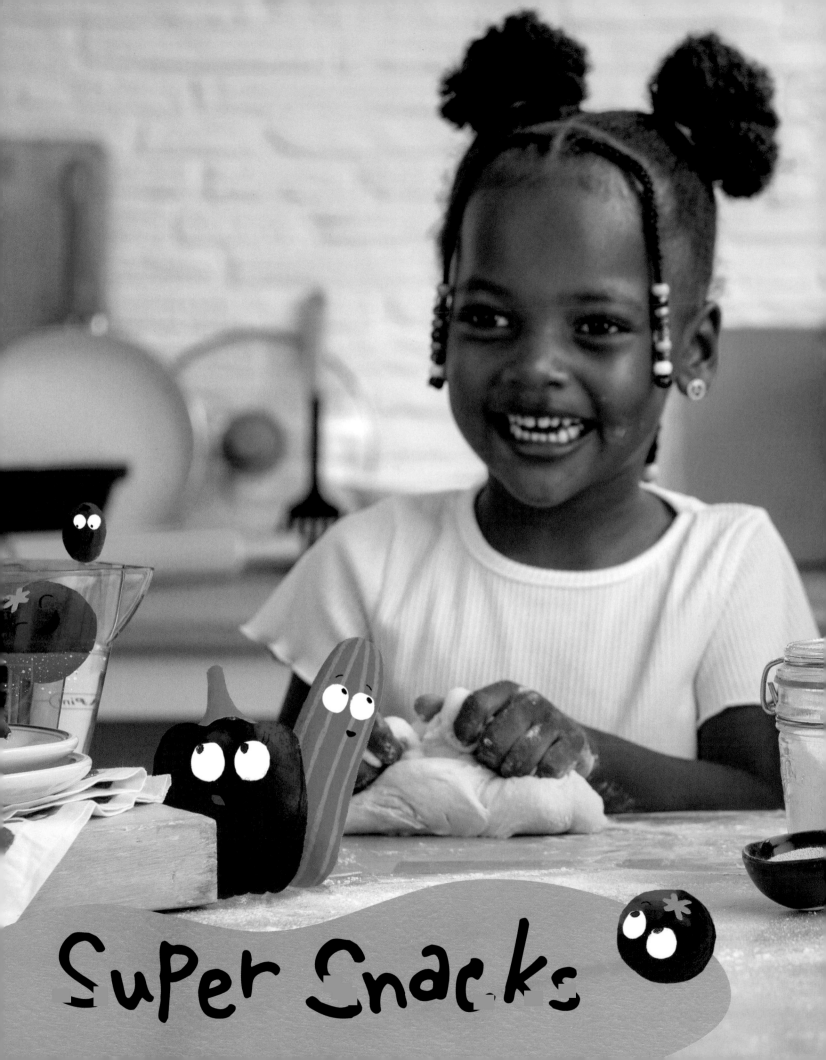

Super Snacks

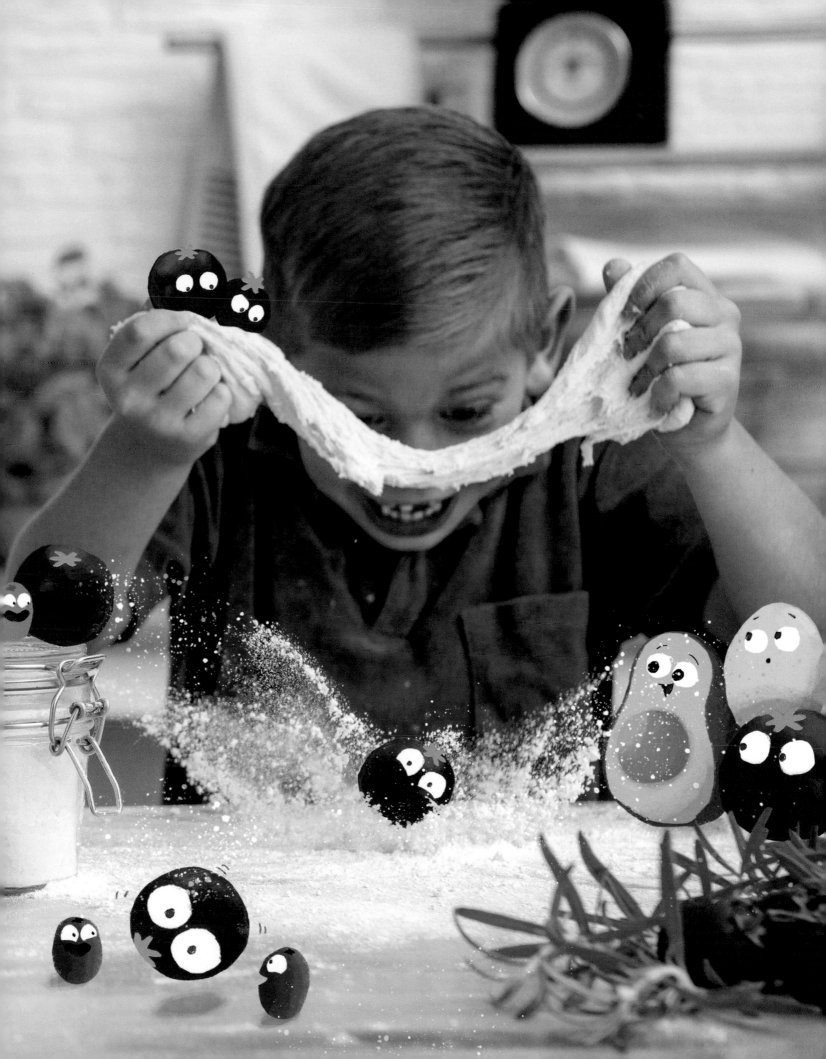

Two-tone sandwiches

Get your cookie cutters out for these simple, fast and super fun sandwiches!

You will need

 6 slices wholemeal bread

 6 slices white bread

 soft butter

 2 eggs

 6 tablespoons mayonnaise

 1 small cooked chicken breast, diced

 2 tablespoons sweetcorn

 2 tablespoons chives, chopped

 2 tablespoons hummus

 ¼ cucumber, thinly sliced

Equipment
Shaped cookie cutters

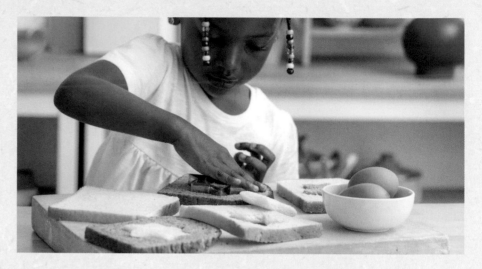

1 Put one slice of brown bread and one slice of white bread on a board. Stamp out a star shape using a cutter from the centre of both slices. Swap the cutout over so you have a white star in a brown slice of bread and a brown star in a white slice of bread. Repeat with the other slices using different shapes.

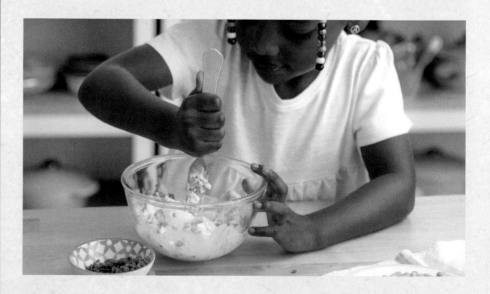

2 Cook the eggs in boiling water for 12 minutes. Cool under cold water, peel and mash in a bowl. Add half the mayonnaise and chives.

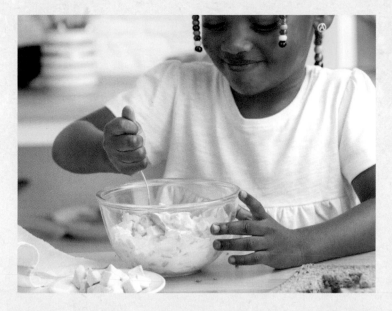

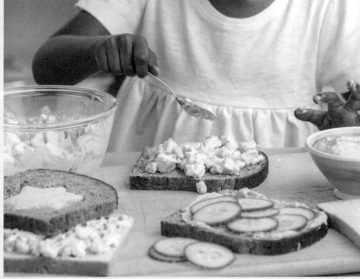

3 Mix the chicken, sweetcorn and the rest of the mayo together in a bowl. Season with salt and pepper. Now spread one side of the bread with butter.

4 Divide the egg filling between two slices, then sandwich together. Repeat with the chicken mixture. For the hummus sandwiches, spoon on hummus and add cucumber before closing the sandwich.

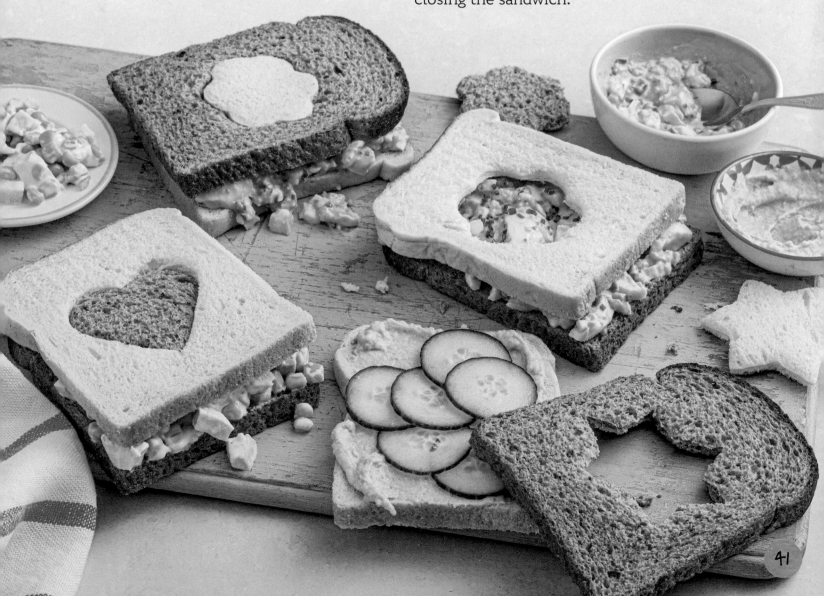

Monster pizzas

Get your cauldron out and round up your little witches and wizards for a monster pizza party!

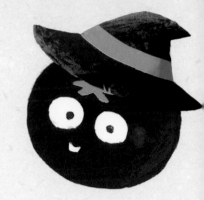

You will need

 325g (11.5 oz) ready-rolled puff pastry

 140g (½ cup) passata

 1 clove garlic, crushed

 1 tablespoon sundried tomato paste

 100g (3.5 oz) grated Mozzarella, plus **100g (3.5 oz)** firm Mozzarella, sliced into strips

 black olives, stoned

 green and red peppers, sliced

 50g (2 oz) sliced ham

 salad leaves

Equipment
9-10cm (3.5"-4") round cutter, baking tray, baking paper

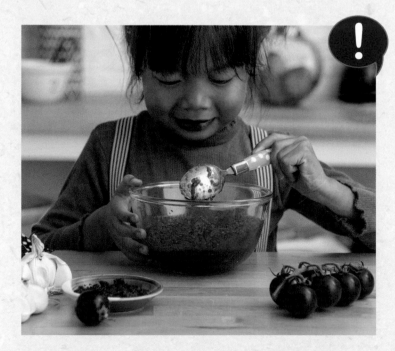

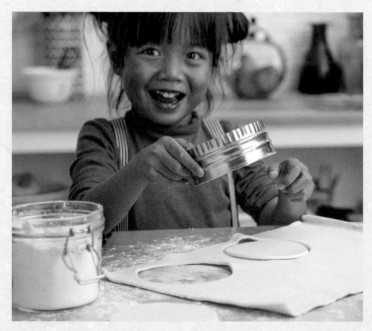

1 Preheat the oven to 200°C (400°F) Fan. Line a large baking sheet with baking paper. Mix the passata, garlic and sundried tomato paste together in a small bowl.

2 Unroll the pastry. Cut out 7 circles using the round cutter. Place on a baking sheet lined with baking paper.

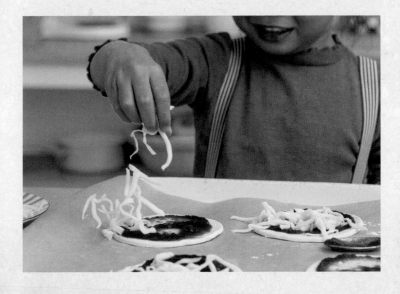

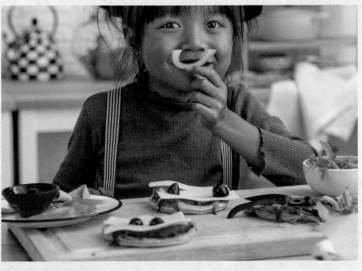

3 Spread the sauce over the bases, sprinkle with grated Mozzarella. Cook in the oven for 18–20 minutes until golden and crisp.

4 Decorate the pizzas to make the monster and mummy faces.

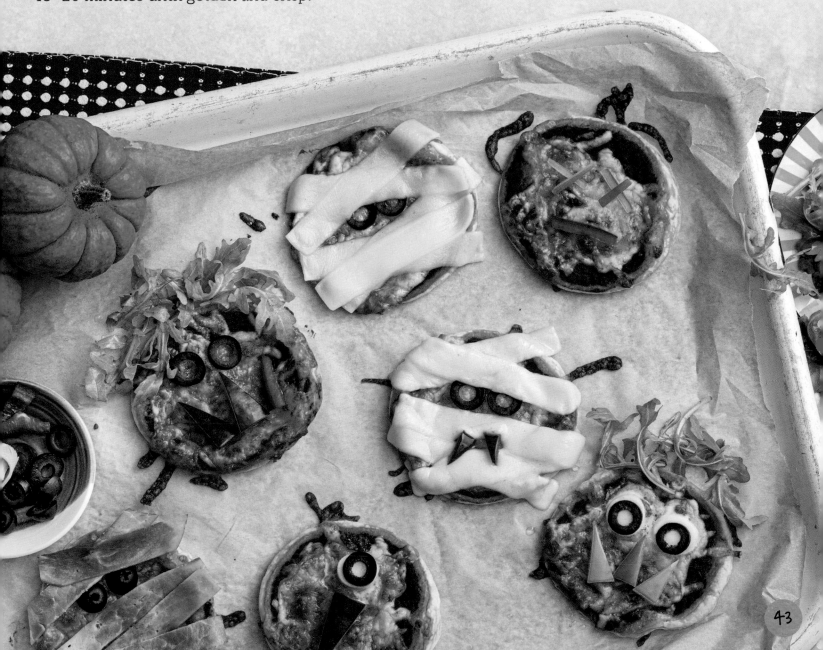

Serves
8

Veggie

Prep time
2 ½ hrs

Cooking
25 mins

Rosemary and tomato focaccia

A delicious bread recipe that's so simple,
kids will love to make it.

You will need

 350g (2 ¾ cups) strong white flour

 2 teaspoons yeast

 ½ teaspoon salt

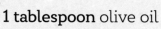 **1 tablespoon** olive oil

 200ml (¾ cup) water

 10 cherry tomatoes

 rosemary sprigs

 1 egg, beaten

 25g (2 tablespoons) Parmesan cheese, grated

 1 clove garlic, crushed

Equipment
Baking dish, baking paper,
cling film, rolling pin

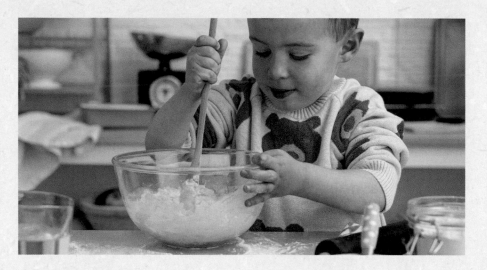

1 Make the dough. Put the flour, yeast, salt, olive oil, water and garlic into a bowl. Mix together using a wooden spoon until the mixture comes together.

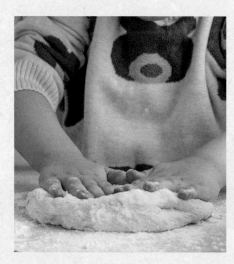

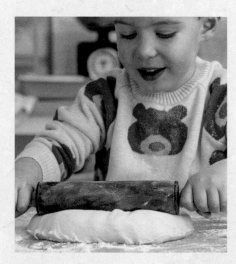

2 Knead into a soft dough on a work surface. Place in an oiled bowl, cover with clingfilm, and leave to rise for 1 ½ hours.

3 Knock back the dough on a work surface. Roll out the dough to a rough rectangle about 40cm (16") long and 25cm (10") wide.

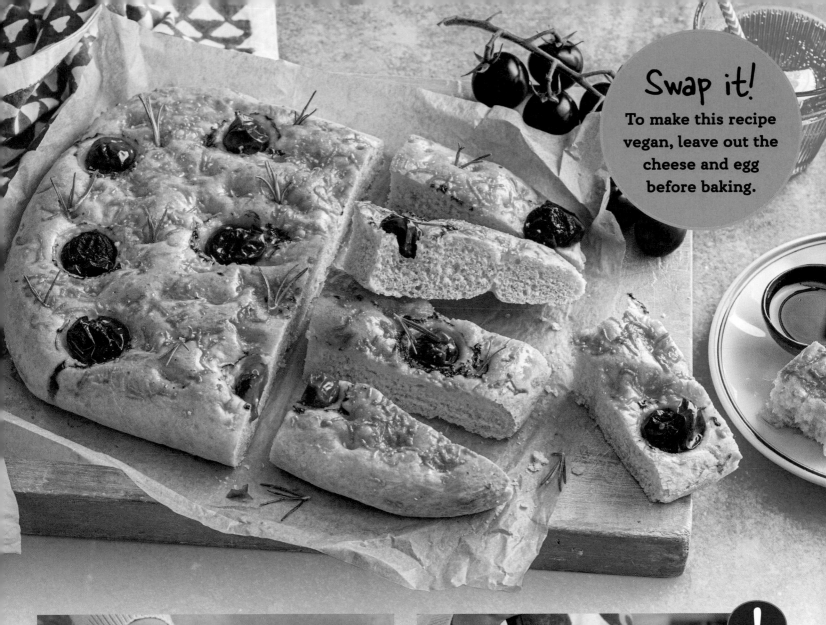

Swap it!
To make this recipe vegan, leave out the cheese and egg before baking.

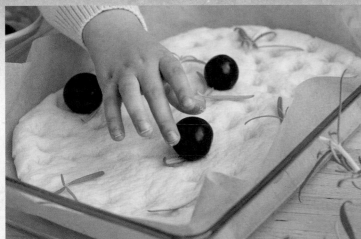

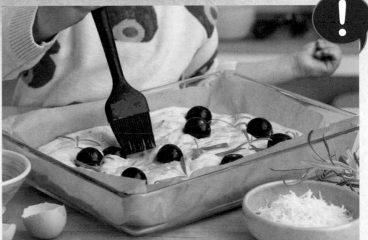

4 Place on a baking dish lined with baking paper. Make holes in the dough. Place the tomatoes on top of the dough and insert sprigs of rosemary. Cover with clingfilm and leave to prove for 40 minutes.

5 Brush with beaten egg and sprinkle with the grated cheese. Preheat the oven to 200°C (400°F) Fan. Bake in the oven for 25 minutes until golden and well risen.

Avocado, Mozzarella and tomato wrap

This is a great lunchtime treat that kids can make all by themselves.

You will need

 2 tortilla wraps

 2 heaped tablespoons fresh pesto

 100g (3.5 oz) cherry tomatoes, quartered

 125g (4.5 oz) Mozzarella ball, diced

 ½ avocado, diced

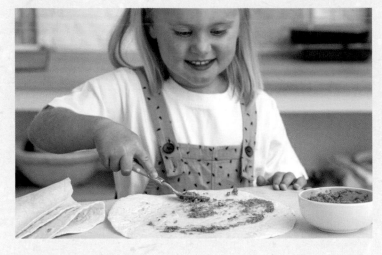

1 Warm the tortilla wraps in the microwave for 10 seconds. Place them on a board and spread the pesto over the wrap.

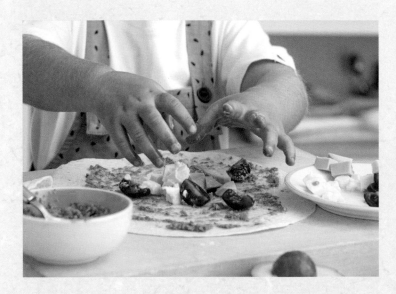

2 Top with the tomatoes, Mozzarella and avocado.

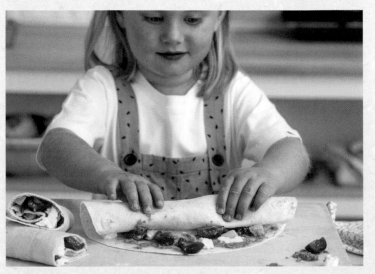

3 Roll up tightly. Slice each wrap in half. Your wrap is ready to serve.

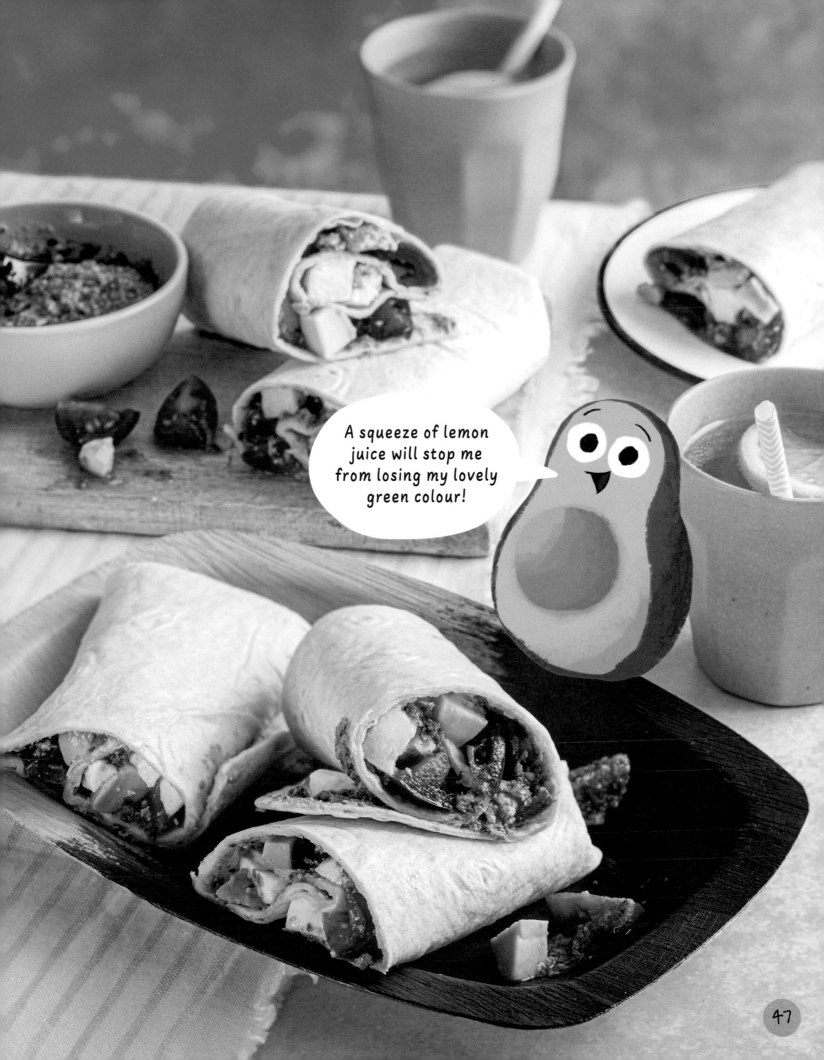

Caterpillar sandwich

This cheeky caterpillar makes the perfect centrepiece for a party spread.

You will need

 8 slices of bread

 soft butter

 4 slices of Gruyere cheese

 4 slices of ham

 1 large tomato

 1 slice of Gruyere cheese

 a little cream cheese

 black olives

 cucumber

 cocktail sticks

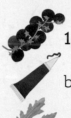 1 cherry tomato

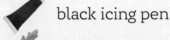 black icing pen

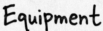 rocket/arugula

Equipment
Small round cookie cutter, small flower cookie cutter

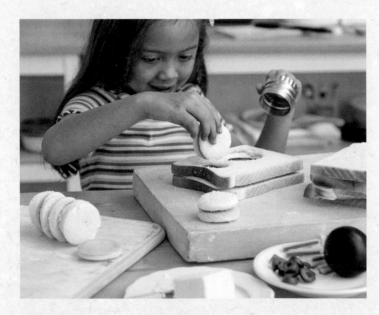

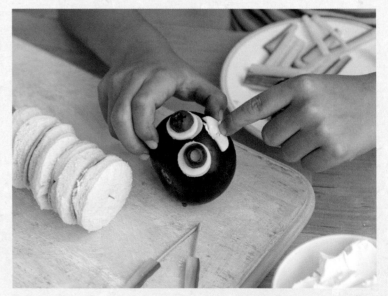

1 Put the slices of bread on a board. Spread with butter. Top four slices with cheese and ham, then sandwich the bread together. Stamp out four small rounds from each sandwich, and arrange on a serving board in a curved shape.

2 Stamp out two small rounds of cheese and black olives for the eyes and a semicircle for the mouth. Stick onto the tomato using a little cream cheese.

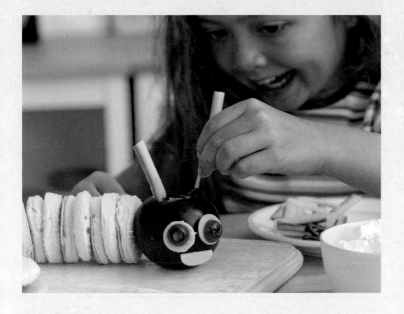

4 Slice the cucumber into two small strips. Insert half a cocktail stick into the cucumber strips, then stick in the top of the tomato to make the antennae.

5 Make a small ladybug out of half a cherry tomato and half a black olive. Add spots using black writing icing.

6 Stamp out cucumber flowers using a cutter. Scatter rocket and cucumber flowers around the caterpillar.

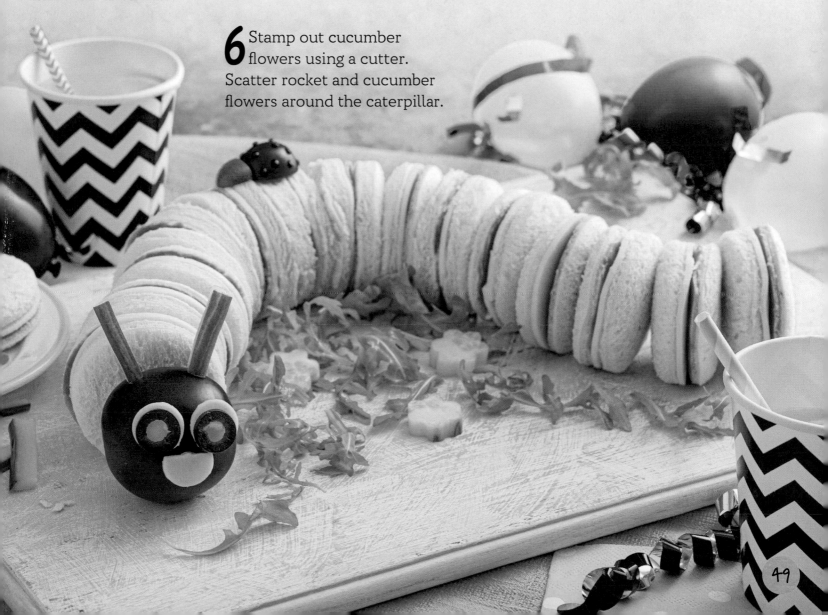

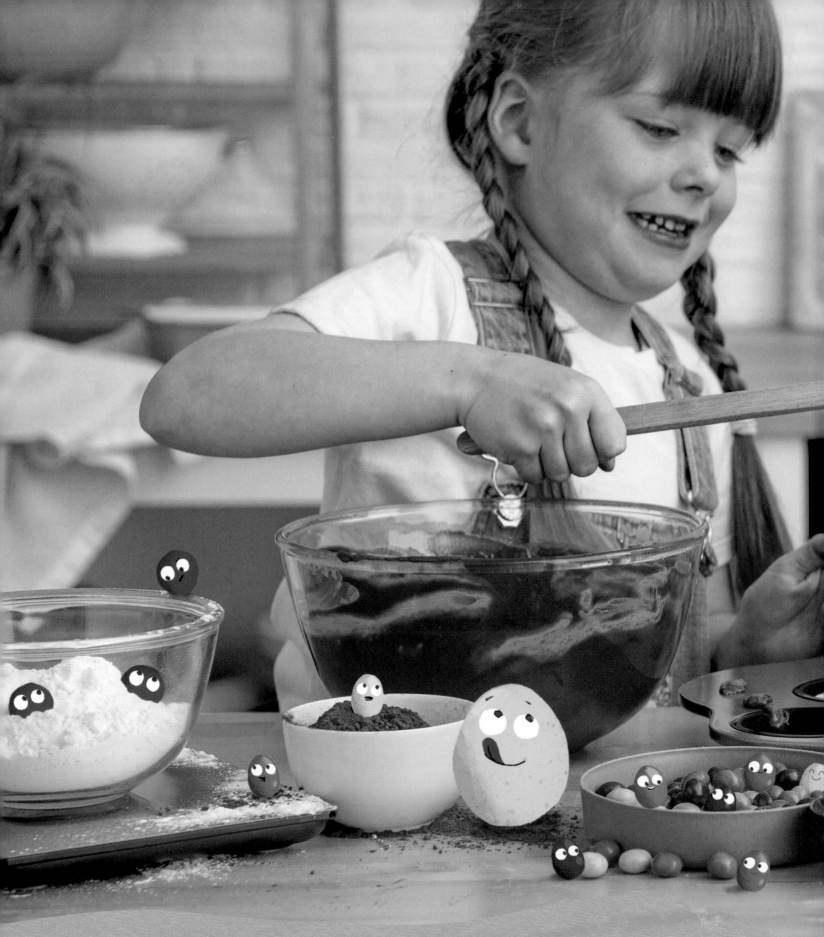

Sweets and Desserts

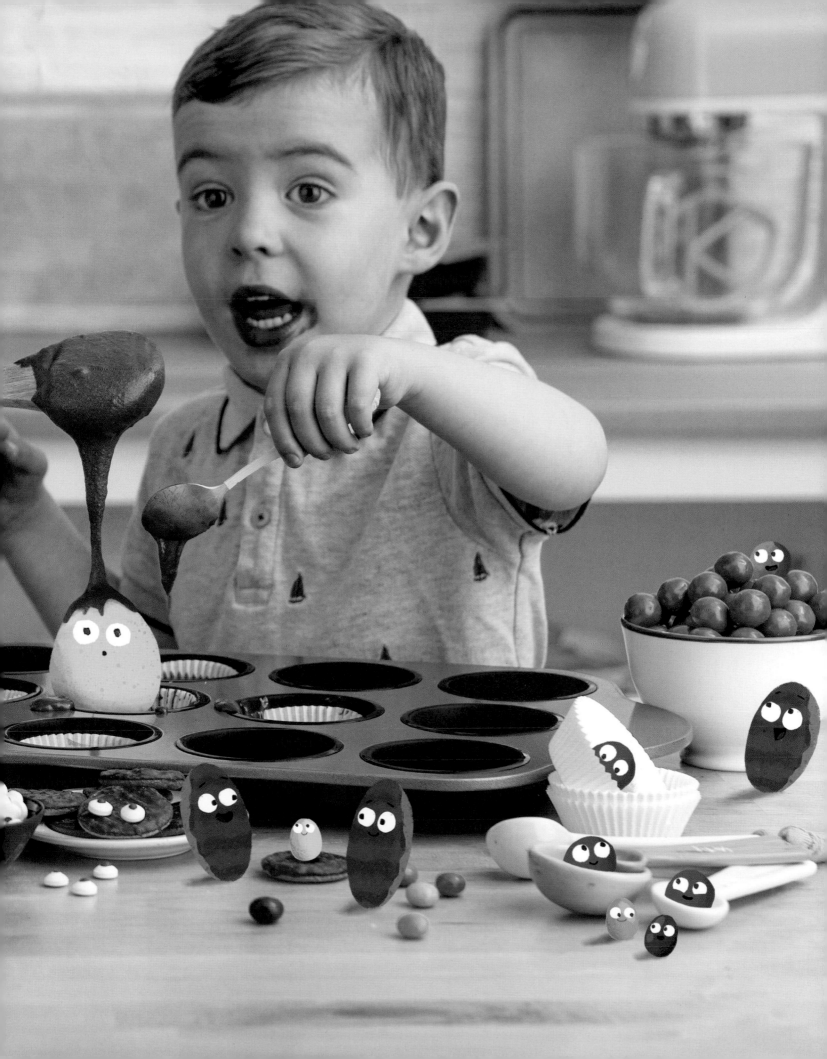

Serves
8

Veggie

Prep time
20mins

Cooking
1hr

Banana and blueberry loaf cake

Slice up this fruit-filled loaf to make a delicious doggy face!

You will need

 150g (⅔ cup) butter, softened

125g (¾ cup) light brown sugar

2 eggs

1 teaspoon vanilla extract

200g (7 oz) overripe bananas, mashed, plus extra slices

 225g (2 cups) self-raising flour

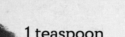 **1 teaspoon** mixed spice

 100g (3.5 oz) blueberries

To decorate

banana

a few blueberries

a few raspberries

Equipment
900g (32 oz) loaf tin, baking paper

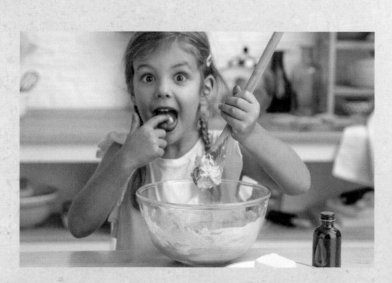

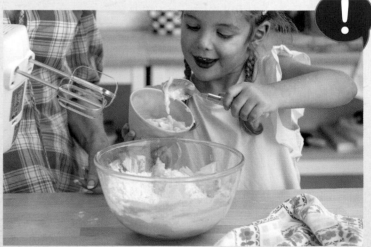

1 Preheat the oven to 160°C (325°F) Fan. Grease and line a loaf tin with non-stick paper. Whisk the butter and sugar together in a mixing bowl until fluffy.

2 Add the eggs, vanilla, bananas, flour and mixed spice. Whisk together using an electric hand whisk.

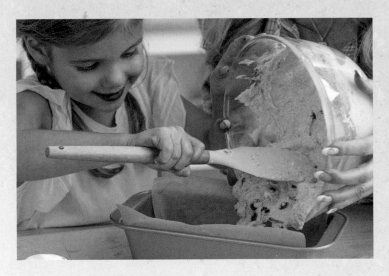

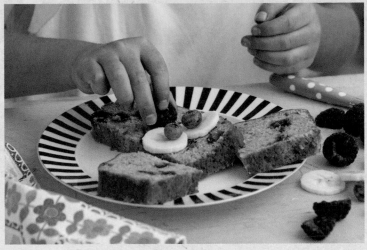

3 Fold in the blueberries and spoon into the loaf tin. Bake in the oven for 50 mins-1 hour until well risen and lightly golden.

4 Slice into slices and arrange on a plate to look like a dog's face and ears. Add banana slices and blueberries for the eyes and nose, and a raspberry for the tongue.

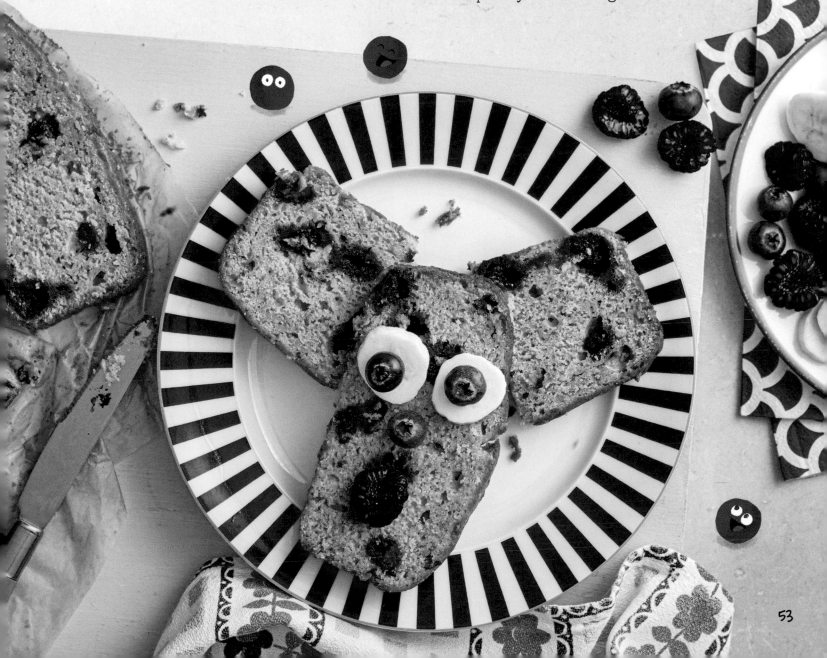

Oreo brownies

These soft and squishy brownies are jazzed up with Oreo cookies.

You will need

250g (**1 cup**) butter

250g (**1 ½ cups**) light brown sugar

4 eggs

2 teaspoons vanilla extract

100g (**1 cup**) cocoa powder

100g (**¾ cup**) plain flour

pinch salt

1 packet Oreos

Equipment

23cm (9") square tin, baking paper

If you like your brownies super-squishy, take them out of the oven a couple of minutes early!

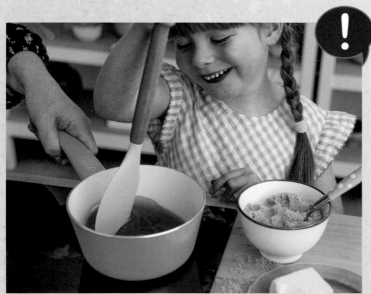

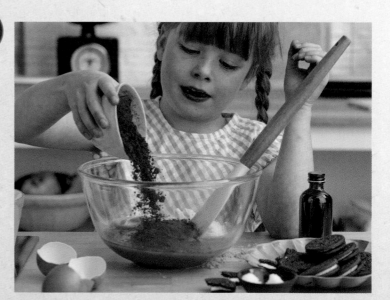

1 Preheat the oven to 180°C (400°F) Fan. Grease and line the square tin with non-stick paper. Put the butter and sugar into a pan and melt on a low heat, or melt the butter and sugar in a bowl over a pan of boiling water.

2 Remove from the heat and add the eggs and vanilla and stir. Add the cocoa powder, flour and salt. Mix well.

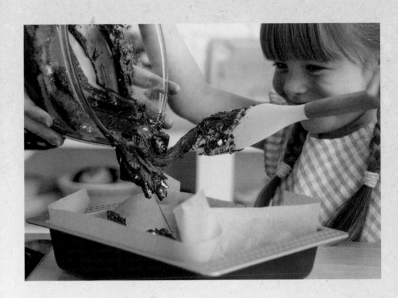 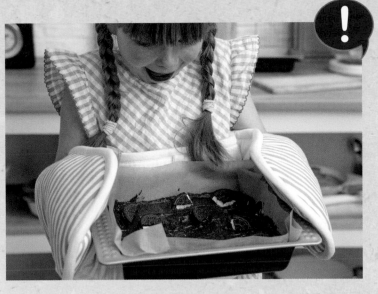

3 Break the cookies into pieces and fold half of the Oreos into the mixture. Pour into the tin. Put the remaining Oreos on top.

4 Bake for 35 minutes until well risen and firm in the centre. Cool on a wire rack. Slice into squares.

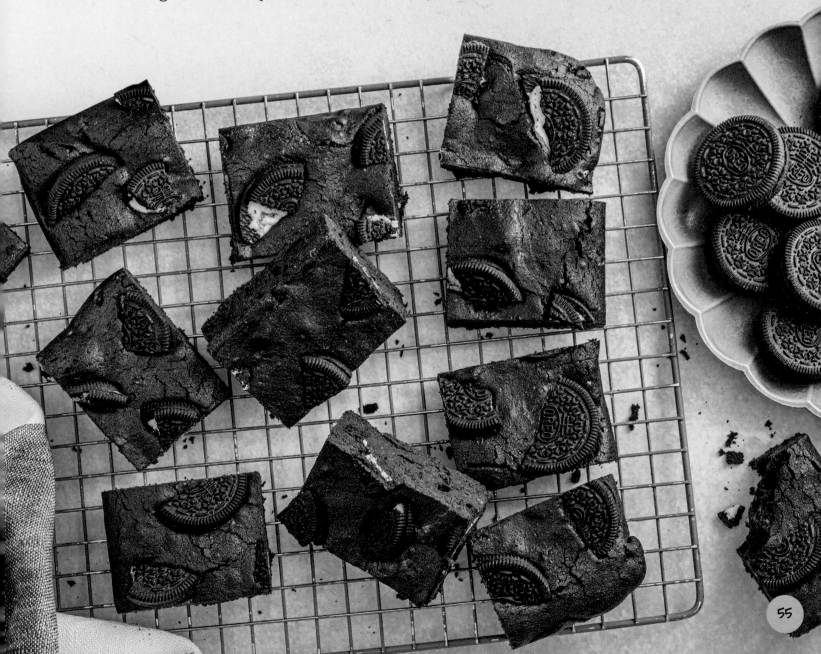

Mother's day cookies

These heart-shaped cookies make the perfect mother's day present. Try not to eat them all first!

You will need

 175g (1 ½ cup) plain flour

 100g (7 tablespoons) chilled butter, cubed

 85g (⅔ cup) icing sugar, plus additional to dust cookies with

 1 teaspoon vanilla extract

 1 egg yolk

 ⅛ teaspoon salt

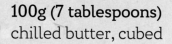 **6 tablespoons** raspberry or strawberry jam

Equipment

Large and small heart-shaped cookie cutters, sieve for dusting with icing sugar, rolling pin, food processor

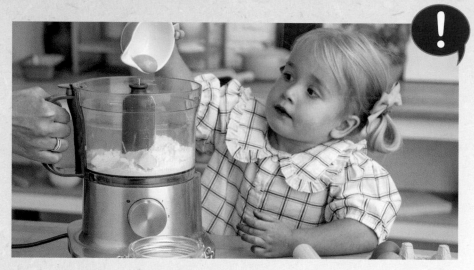

1 Put the flour, butter, sugar, salt, vanilla and egg yolk in a food processor. Dribble in a tablespoon of water, and whizz until the mix comes together to form a dough. Place onto a work surface, and knead briefly to bring together. Now wrap in cling film, and chill for 20 minutes.

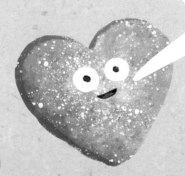

Why not bake all the little hearts you have left over from cutting out the centres? They make cute mini cookies like me!

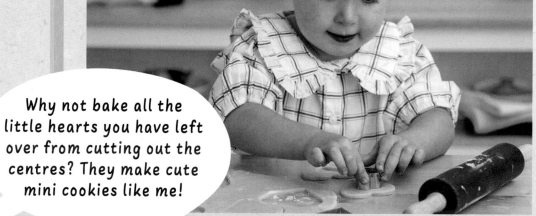

2 Once chilled, roll out on a floured surface using a rolling pin and cut 30 heart shapes. Using a smaller heart cutter, cut a small heart in the middle of 15 of the biscuits.

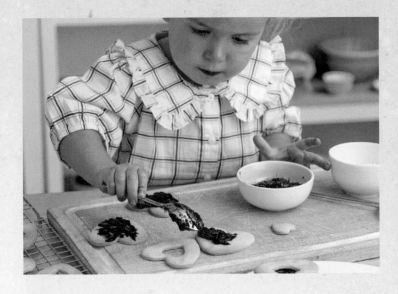

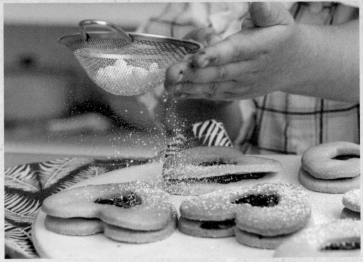

3 Bake in an oven preheated to 160°C (325°F) Fan for 12 minutes, or until light golden brown. When completely cool, spread some jam on the complete hearts, leaving a small border around the edge.

4 Carefully place each heart with the middle cut out on top of a jam-covered heart, and lightly press together. Dust the cookies lightly with icing sugar using a small sieve.

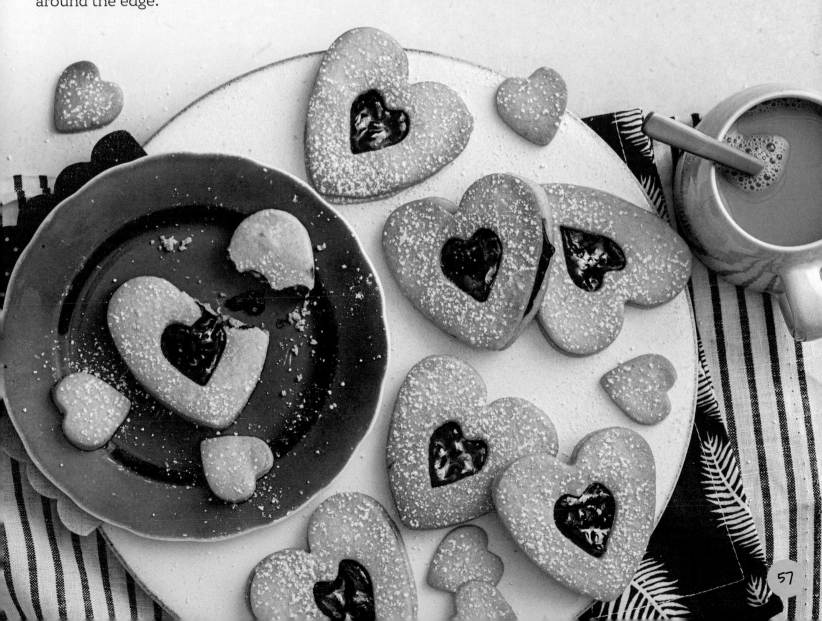

Crêpes with Nutella and banana

You can add whatever you like to these classic pancakes – I love folding in Nutella and banana slices.

Ask an adult to try flipping these pancakes in the pan!

You will need

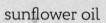

100g (¾ cup) plain flour

2 large eggs

225ml (1 cup) milk

sunflower oil

Nutella spread

4 bananas, sliced

mixed fruit

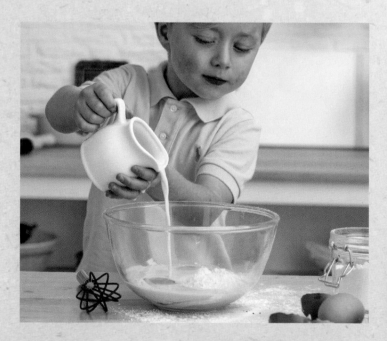

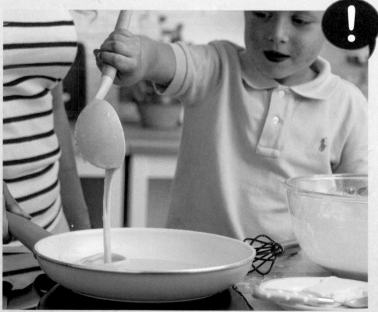

1 Measure the flour into a bowl. Add the eggs and a quarter of the milk. Whisk to a smooth consistency, then whisk in the remaining milk to make a smooth batter.

2 Heat a tablespoon of oil in a small frying pan. Spoon a small amount of the batter into the centre of the pan, and tilt to make a thin layer covering the base.

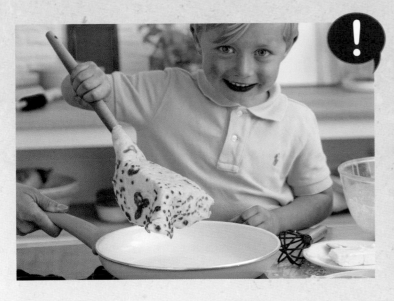

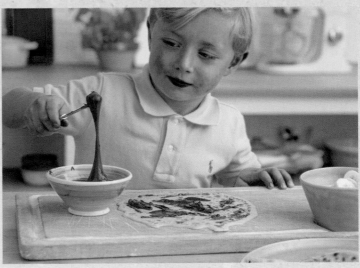

3 Heat for 2-3 minutes until the batter is set. Loosen the sides of the crêpe using a palette knife. Flip over and cook on the other side until pale golden. Place on a plate. Repeat the method to make 10 thin crêpes.

4 Place one crêpe on a board. Spread a tablespoon of Nutella over the surface. Add slices of bananas. Fold in half and half again to make a triangle shape. Repeat with the remaining crêpes.

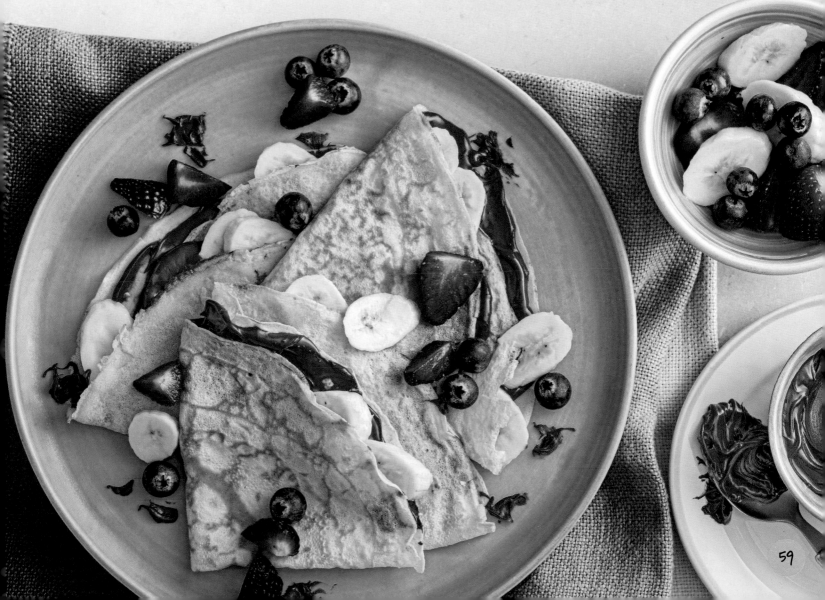

Teddy bear cupcakes

These cute little cupcakes are perfect for a teddy bears' picnic!

You will need

 3 eggs

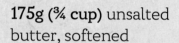 175g (¾ cup) unsalted butter, softened

 150g (1 ¼ cups) self-raising flour

 25g (¼ cup) cocoa powder

 175g (1 cup) caster sugar

 2 tablespoons milk

 1 teaspoon baking powder

For the frosting

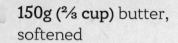 150g (⅔ cup) butter, softened

 300g (2 ¼ cups) icing sugar, sieved

 2 tablespoons milk

3 tablespoons cocoa powder, sieved

To decorate

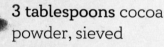 white and milk chocolate buttons

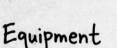 12 Maltesers/Whoppers

6 mini Jaffa Cakes or similar cookies

24 edible eyes

Equipment
Muffin tin, muffin cases, piping bag and fluted nozzle (optional)

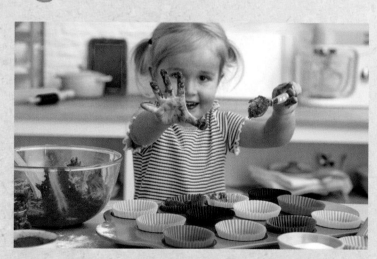

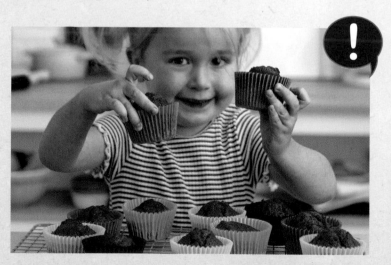

1 Preheat the oven to 160°C (325°F) Fan. Line a 12 hole muffin tin with paper cases. Measure all of the cupcake ingredients into a large mixing bowl and whisk until smooth. Divide the mixture between the 12 muffin cases.

2 Bake for 20 to 25 minutes until well risen and firm to the touch. Leave to cool on a wire rack.

60

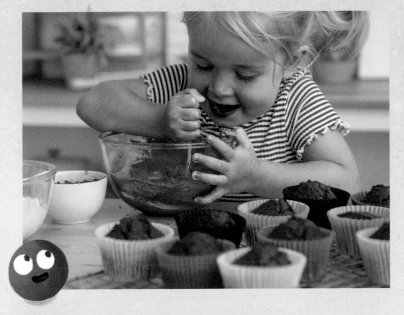

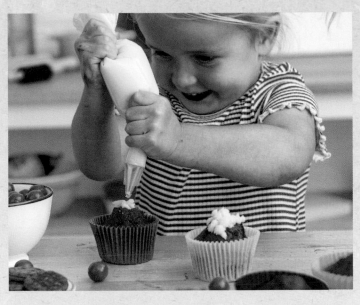

3 For the frosting, mix the butter, icing sugar and milk together in a large bowl Whisk until light and fluffy. Divide the mixture into two bowls. Add the cocoa powder to one bowl and mix well.

4 Spoon into a piping bag with a fluted nozzle if piping the icing – or you can spread the icing onto the cupcakes with a spatula.

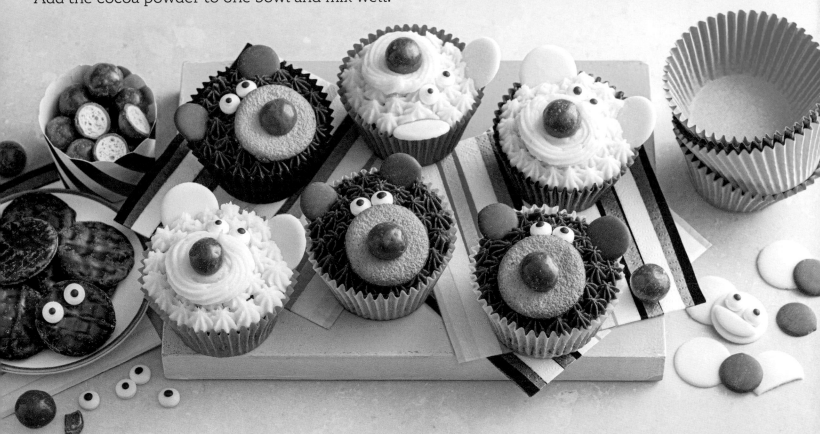

5 For the 6 milk chocolate cupcakes, pipe or spread the chocolate icing on top for the teddy bear's face. Put a Jaffa Cake and a Malteser on top for the nose. Add two milk chocolate buttons for the ears, and two edible eyes.

6 For the white chocolate cupcakes, pipe or spread the icing on 6 of the cupcakes. Insert two white chocolate buttons for the ears and a Malteser for the nose. Add edible eyes to finish.

Gingerbread friends

It's so easy to make these gingerbread people,
and it's fun to 'dress' them with any decorations you like.

You will need

140g (⅔ cup) butter, softened

80g (½ cup) brown sugar

50g (2 ½ tablespoons) golden syrup

50g (2 ½ tablespoons) black treacle

½ egg, beaten

150g (1 ¼ cups) plain flour

150g (1 ¼ cups) self-raising flour

2 teaspoons cinnamon

2 teaspoons ginger

1 teaspoon mixed spice

½ teaspoon allspice

pinch salt

To decorate

M&M's

icing pens

edible eyes

Equipment
Hand whisk, baking sheet, baking paper,
gingerbread person cutter, rolling pin

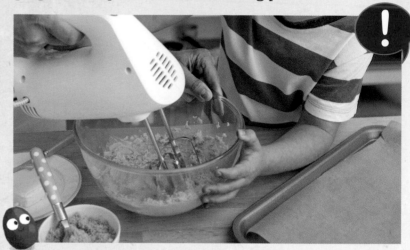

1 Preheat the oven 170°C (340°F) Fan. Line two baking sheets with non-stick baking paper. Whisk the butter and sugar in a mixing bowl, until light and fluffy.

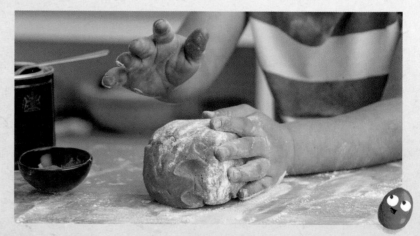

2 Add the syrup and treacle and egg. Mix well. Add the flours, spices and salt. Mix again until you have a soft dough. Wrap in clingfilm and chill the dough in the fridge for 30 minutes.

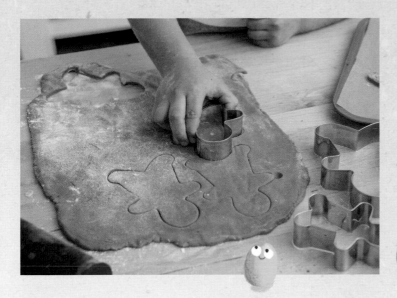
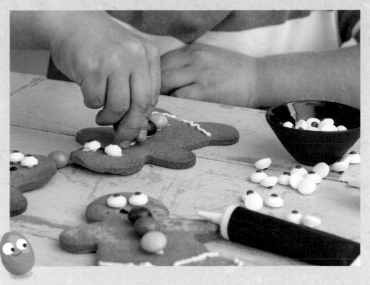

3 Roll out the dough on a floured work surface. Stamp out 20 gingerbread shapes. Place on the baking sheets.

4 Bake for about 15 minutes until lightly golden and firm in the middle. Cool on a wire rack. Decorate the cookies to make people using the M&M's, icing pens and edible eyes.

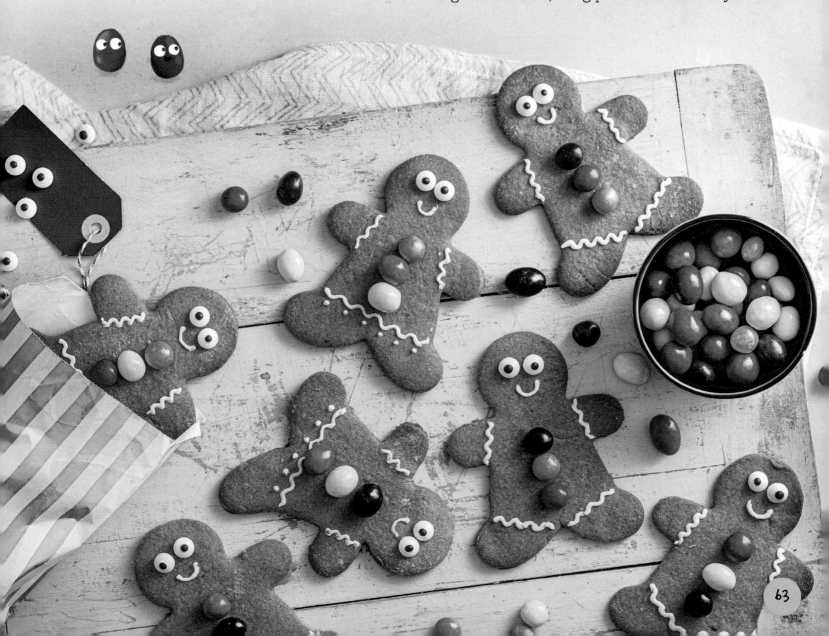

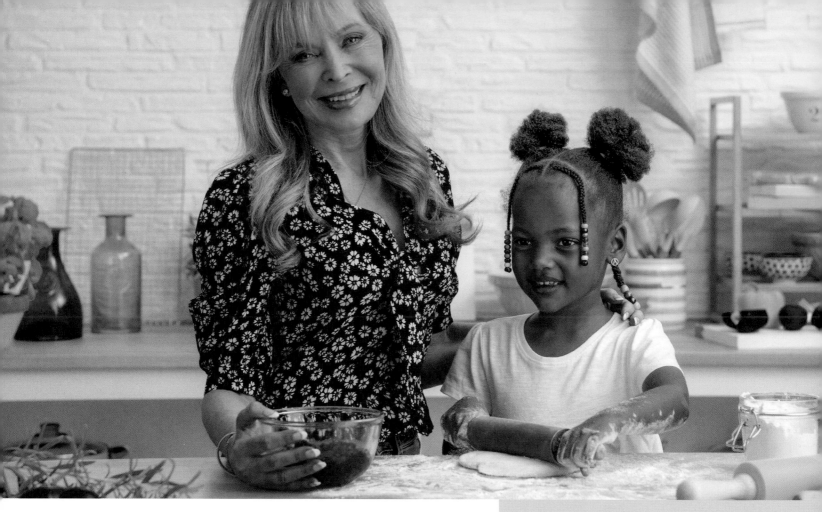

About
Annabel Karmel

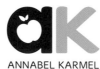
ANNABEL KARMEL

With expertise spanning over 30 years, London-born mother of three Annabel Karmel reigns as the UK's no. 1 children's cookery author, best selling international author, and a world-leading expert on devising delicious, nutritious meals for babies, children and families.

Since launching her revolutionary cookbook for babies - *The Complete Baby & Toddler Meal Planner* in 1991 - a feeding 'bible', which has sold over 6 million copies and become the 2nd bestselling non-fiction hardback of all time, Annabel has raised millions of families on her recipes.

My First Cookbook marks Annabel's 50th published title. Annabel's vision has always been to ensure every child gets the nutrition they need for their development and long-term health, and her unique, tasty recipes have made her a true pioneer in her field.

Annabel has a big social media community, sharing new recipes and advice every day. Her award-winning *Baby & Toddler Recipe App* is jam-packed with 650+ recipes, plus tasty new ideas every week. Paired with meal planners, shopping lists, helpful guides, and more, it's a kitchen essential for busy families.

Annabel's trusty cookbook-inspired meals for toddlers and kids can also be discovered in supermarkets. Low in salt and a tasty way towards their 5 a day, her ready-to-go recipes are the perfect fuel for daily adventures. Discover them in the chilled and frozen aisles and online. Annabel's menus are also served-up across world-leading hotels, leisure resorts and nurseries.

In 2006, Annabel received an MBE in the Queen's Birthday Honours for her outstanding work in the field of child nutrition. From kitchen table to global stage, Annabel is loved and trusted all over the world for raising healthy, happy eaters.

Annabel Karmel's No.1 Rated Recipe App

Looking for mealtime inspiration for your baby, toddler or child? Annabel's award-winning recipe app is filled with over 650 simple and delicious ideas, PLUS new recipes every week.

With lots of tasty ideas and helpful tools, it's a kitchen essential for happy, healthy mealtimes.

Scan me!

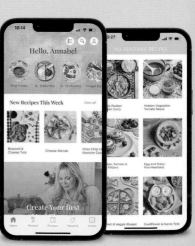

Available on the App Store

GET IT ON Google Play

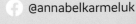

📷 @annabelkarmel   f @annabelkarmeluk

annabelkarmel.com   📌 @annabelkarmel